D0129060

THE ART OF SEXUAL
INTIMACY

Truly intimate sex can be a reality. This book explains why more and more people — men and women — are aspiring to deeper levels of sexual intimacy and then shows how you can enhance your one-to-one relationship in this way.

Intimacy means different things to different people and involves an infinite range of emotions and behaviors. In Part One, Dr Stanway explains that before we can become really intimate with our partner we have to get to know ourselves. This involves becoming aware of our own attitudes to intimacy and how they were formed in childhood. Drawing heavily on his professional experience as a therapist, he delves deeply into the complex, fascinating and controversial research that has been undertaken in this core area.

Sex can be enjoyed on many different levels. Intimate sex, however, is the ultimate love-making experience and in Part Two Dr Stanway describes the many ways in which couples can achieve this. In his terms, sexual intimacy is part of a couple's life-style together; enhances their value to each other; can be varied according to the situation; has limitless horizons; copes well with failure; includes heart and soul as well as body; tends to improve with time and is a lifetime's investment.

But no matter how much you and your partner love one another or know the theory nothing happens by magic to make you more intimate. Intimacy takes time and effort. Practical exercises for building your intimate life together are given in Part Three.

This topical book will fascinate, inform and stimulate. With its clear, practical advice and beautiful, sensitive color photography, THE ART OF SEXUAL INTIMACY is essential reading for every couple wanting to enhance their relationship year after year.

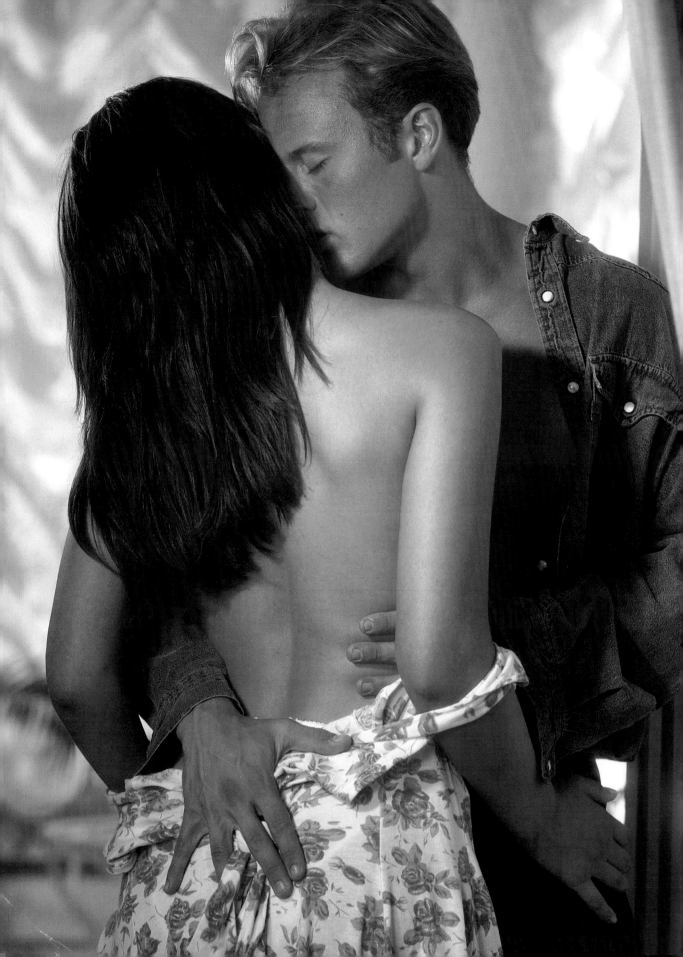

THE ART OF SEXUAL INTIMACY

Dr Andrew Stanway

Photography by Ralph Medland

Carroll & Graf Publishers, Inc.
New York

Text copyright © Dr Andrew Stanway 1993
This edition copyright © Eddison Sadd Editions 1993

The right of Dr Andrew Stanway to be
identified as the author of the work has been
asserted by him in accordance with the
Copyright, Designs and Patents Act 1988.

All rights reserved.

First published in the United States in 1993
by Carroll & Graf Publishers, Inc.

Second printing 1993

Carroll & Graf Publishers, Inc.
260 Fifth Avenue
New York, NY 10001

**Library of Congress
Cataloging-in-Publication Data**
is available on request from
Carroll & Graf.

ISBN 0-88184-925-1

AN EDDISON · SADD EDITION
Edited, designed and produced by
Eddison Sadd Editions Limited
St Chad's Court
146B King's Cross Road
London WC1X 9DH

Make-up and stylist Claire Stevens
Phototypeset in Usherwood ITC Book
by Dorchester Typesetting,
Dorchester, England
Origination by Columbia Offset, Singapore
Printed and bound by Dai Nippon, Hong Kong

CONTENTS

INTRODUCTION

Don't walk in front of me, I may not follow. Don't walk behind me, I may not lead. Walk beside me and just be my friend.
ANON

Sexual intimacy is something to which most of us aspire. In my experience as a psychosexual and marital therapist, however, I have found that many people focus unrealistically on the 'sexual' aspects of their relationships and far too little on 'intimacy'. Most of us start off as a couple fondly hoping that things will get better and better. Reality soon dawns, however. Once the initial fizz has gone out of the relationship, it becomes clear that we have to settle down and learn more about ourselves and our partners if we are to survive, let alone thrive, as lovers.

Today's world is somewhat hostile to couples. Much of what masquerades as intimacy in popular culture is pure sham. This leaves countless millions of individuals disappointed with their one-to-one relationships which, in a world run on disposable lines, are soon discarded. The emotional, financial and human costs of this approach can hardly be measured.

Listening, as I do, to couples sharing their innermost hopes, fears, dreams and aspirations, I cannot but come to the conclusion that most of us pair with good intent, certain that we will not go the way of our parents, friends and acquaintances. Somehow we can make things work. Love will conquer all.

Alas, this expectation, like so many others in one-to-one relationships, is totally unfounded. Some people make terrible partner choices; others choose excellent mates and then foul things up; yet others, seeking perfection, run from partner to partner, unconsciously working through their own pains while blaming the other person for their own failings. Corpses of pair-bonding litter the modern landscape.

Over the last thirty years or so it has become a popular expectation that couples should try to make their lives more fulfilling by enhancing their sexual knowledge and prowess. Certainly this can do no harm but equally it is not the answer to making relationships work, in or out of bed. And in an age of AIDS it is perhaps even more important for anyone in a loving one-to-one relationship to try to make it work. Sexual dalliances are less attractive now that they carry such health risks and more people seem intent on saving and improving what they have.

In a world in which sex is now the legitimate subject of dinner-party and playground discussion, open communication is usually much less fraught than it was even twenty years ago. However, though some people can readily talk about their orgasms, contraceptive practices, sexually transmitted diseases, or whatever, few are nearly as forthcoming when talking about intimacy. When I discuss intimacy with my patients they nearly always assume that I mean something physical and probably sexual. Indeed the word intimacy has become inextricably linked with genital expressions of sex. Yet anyone who pauses to think for a moment knows that babies and children can have an intimate relationship with their parents; that adults who have no sexual connection can share truly intimate lives; and so on.

Because of this confusion I have divided *The Art of Sexual Intimacy* into three sections. The first is by far the most extensive and deals with intimacy in its many forms. This is the foundation stone on which any meaningful sexual relationship is built. The second part looks at actual genital intimacy; and the third outlines many skills we can learn if we are to develop our intimate life together as a couple.

But intimacy, in the way that I define it, cannot simply be mastered in one day – like learning how to make an omelette. It is part of a much bigger journey that enriches and enhances our whole life together as a couple. The essence of the journey I will outline is that it leads to a more aware and conscious, as opposed to unaware and unconscious, relationship. No matter what you currently do or do not do sexually; no matter how much pleasure you experience; no matter what your starting point, you will find that following this book through and trying to bring its ideas into your life will increase your sexual pleasure and fulfilment in a way that nothing else ever has or can.

So what do we have to do to become more aware and more conscious? First of all it involves accepting that a relationship is not simply about two people coming together in a haphazard way to be friends and have sex, but that it is also a way in which we unconsciously choose to heal our deepest childhood wounds. Secondly, as we become conscious, we learn more about our *self* and accept that this is the only knowledge worth having. The more we focus on our lover, the less we learn about ourselves and the less able we are to be totally intimate. This journey also involves taking responsibility for communicating our needs and desires to our partner rather than leaving things to chance. You will begin to be aware of the traps that are laid for you by your unconscious and therefore become more able to bypass them. This, in turn, leads to a more realistic and accurate image of yourself and your partner and an ability to separate his or her business from yours, thus reducing conflict.

As we become more aware, we start to see our partner's needs and wishes as valuable in their own right, just like ours. Unconscious couples assume that their partner is there to service them in some way. Conscious couples can put themselves to one side when necessary and be there just for their partner, not out of duty but from unconditional love. But perhaps the key feature of the conscious relationship is that it enables us to come to an understanding of our dark side, the underbelly we normally try to hide from ourselves, and certainly from our partner. In a loving, intimate relationship there are no actors, only real people being themselves and loved for it. There are few situations in life that allow us to explore our dark side and still feel safe and loved. A one-to-one sexual partnership, however, provides us with a potentially ideal opportunity to do this. The rewards and joys of truly intimate sex give us the freedom and confidence to tread the minefield involved in learning about ourselves and our lover.

The Art of Sexual Intimacy is not just a book about how to have a better sex life. Few of my patients ever get far on this journey if they have not learned how to be more intimate outside the bedroom. The essence of this book could be summed up by a maxim I have heard from many people over the years: look after the relationship and the sex will look after itself.

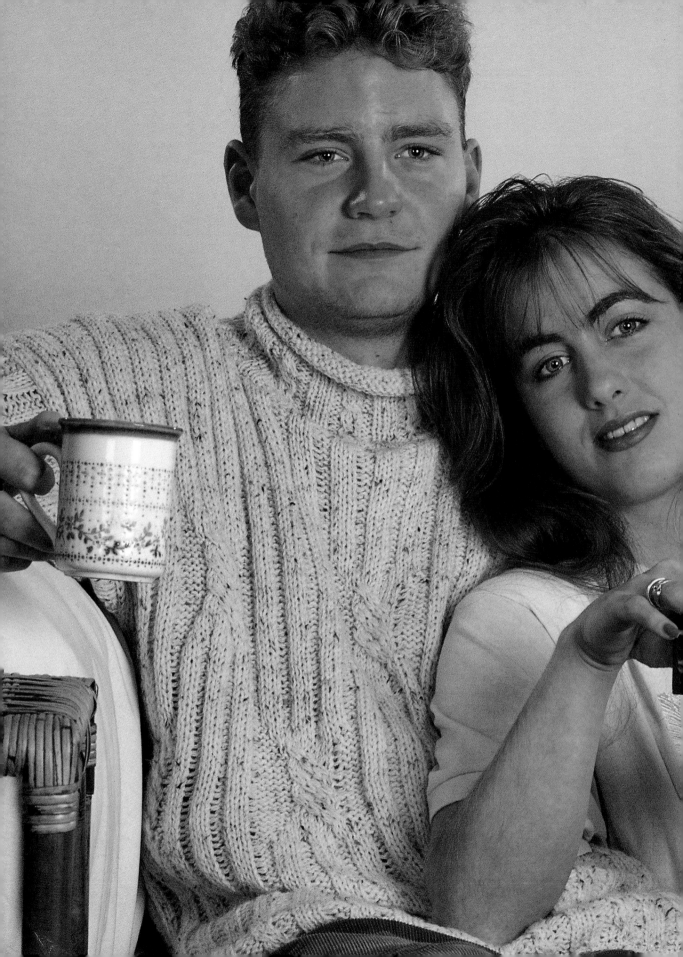

WHAT IS INTIMACY?

Intimacy means many different things to different people. Some see it as 'women's work' yet many men crave more real intimacy in their lives than they currently experience. Love, closeness and intimacy are often confused, as if they were the same thing, which they are not. Most of us are somewhat baffled that we seem to have teamed up with someone who is so different from ourselves. Modern relationships are redefining dependency, personal freedom and commitment and all of these force us to rethink what we mean by intimacy. These areas, and many more, are the subject of Part One.

The word intimacy comes from the Latin *intima*, meaning inner or innermost. *Webster's Dictionary* defines intimate as 'belonging to or characterizing one's deepest nature; suggesting informal warmth or privacy; of a very personal or private nature'. But ask 100 people what they mean by it and you will get as many different answers. Intimacy is an intensely subjective experience and any individual's definition will vary from time to time. To some it immediately means sex; to others, being close; and to yet others, some sort of soul-to-soul connection.

Intimacy, in the way I use the word, means being able to contact our innermost selves. This is not the same as having insight or being introspective. These things involve looking at ourselves, which is no bad thing, but intimacy involves more than this. It is an experience rather than an intellectual endeavour. Such intimacy takes place in the presence of another, usually a human being. As we shall see, however, some people are more able to be intimate with nature, animals or even inanimate objects than they are with people.

At some primitive, biological level we all seek intimacy with the universe around us, yet Western culture has tended to lose touch with this deep connection with the cosmos. As a result, many people now claim that the most important sort of intimacy is that which they experience with another person; the intimacy of becoming aware of themselves in the same space as someone else who is being similarly open. Viewed in this way, being intimate is not only one of the most valuable human experiences but also one of the most courageous. Opening oneself up in the presence of *another* takes courage, but in the presence of *oneself* can call for heroism greater than that required in any other sphere of life. Because it demands such bravery, many of us never even attempt it, preferring to fight shy of really knowing ourselves, particularly in the presence of someone we love.

So far I have hardly mentioned sex. This is because intimacy looked at in the way I have just outlined does not necessarily have anything directly to do with sex. In our culture, however, the individual with whom we are most likely to make this courageous journey is commonly our one-to-one, pair-bonded, special partner. For many of us, this is also the individual with whom we have an exclusive, or near-exclusive, sexual agreement. As a result, intimacy and sex are seen to go together. In reality, it is possible to be truly intimate with an individual with whom we have no sexual connection. Many good friends know this to be true. However, the combination of intimacy and sex is so powerful that couples who enjoy both within their relationship have the advantage of greater potential for growth as each enhances the effects of the other.

As a working therapist, many of the people I see who complain of 'sex problems' are in fact plagued by 'intimacy dis-ease'. They have never experienced intimacy; do not know what it is; cannot create it; and look to sex as some sort of way to obtain it. They feel closest to their partner when making love and may even experience some sort of transcendent spiritual oneness from time to time, so they crave more sex to re-create this blissful state. The fact that equal but different bliss can be obtained in an ongoing way as a part of their non-sexual life seems unlikely at first, but it becomes real as they explore the lifelong journey involved in getting to know themselves.

What Intimacy Means

I hope that you have been able to identify with much of what I have outlined here in defining intimacy. Perhaps it would now be helpful, however, to look at how intimacy reveals itself in the practicalities of our daily lives.

BEING SPECIAL TO SOMEBODY

We all want to be special to somebody. To feel loved and wanted seems to be a basic human necessity. No matter how many people we surround ourselves with in our work and play, most of us have a craving for that one-to-one specialness that only another significant human being can bring.

HAVING SOMEONE WITH WHOM WE CAN BE OURSELVES

Knowing ourselves to be imperfect, as we all do at some deeply unconscious level, it takes courage to be open and therefore vulnerable with another. The trust that this requires, if we are not to be abused, calls for someone who will be there for us and accept us for what we are, warts and all. This universal desire to be accepted probably dates back to the cradle. Human infants are vulnerable for much longer than the young of other animal species. They are at serious risk if abandoned in that early stage of life when they cannot feed, protect, shelter, or care for themselves. My work with regression therapies of various kinds teaches me that deep down in all of us is the fear, even the horror, that we might be so unacceptable that we could be abandoned and left to die. The 'death' we fear in adult life is, of course, not so much physical as spiritual and emotional.

SHARING LIFE WITH SOMEONE WITH WHOM WE CAN JUST 'BE'

In the hurly-burly of modern life most of us spend our time 'doing' rather than 'being'. An intimate relationship, however, does not rely on us doing things together; its value is in allowing us simply to 'be'. Couples who know this sort of intimacy can feel such togetherness and even be aware of their own depths just by being in the same space as their beloved. Many such people claim that it hardly matters what they are talking about or doing, as the feelings of sharing the same space are enough. Perhaps this is all many of us need to reassure ourselves that we are not condemned to a life of existential loneliness.

A SAFE HAVEN

Most of us need at least one person who can provide a sanctuary for us from the competitiveness and harshness of modern life. Such a place where we can shelter safely from the storms of life is an important feature of the intimate life.

'BATTLING' WITH SOMEONE AS WE WORK ON OUR UNCONSCIOUS SHADOW

Most of us unconsciously pair-bond with someone who enables us to work on our deepest wounds and pains (see page 35). If we were to pair with someone just like ourselves, we would never grow. This is because there would not be enough difference to create the necessary levels of friction between us. It is almost impossible for most of us to work out our own salvation totally alone, though yogic masters can probably achieve this using their particular methods. The vast majority of us need someone we can trust; someone who loves and respects us enough to allow us to work through our pains from the past. In an intimate relationship not only do we have the advantage of doing this alongside someone who cares, but we also have someone uniquely equipped to mirror our psychic shadow because he or she is both mirror *and* shadow. For more on this, see page 35.

HAVING A SEXUAL SOUL MATE

If, as I assert, really good sex takes place only between intimates, then one of the most important parts of our intimate life together will be the exclusive expression of our spirituality through sexual connection (see page 84).

SETTING AN EXAMPLE FOR OUR CHILDREN

For those who choose marriage and children, the intimate life provides a seed bed in which the next generation can experience intimacy. They will learn from the love their parents show them and each other. This subject is considered at greater length on page 82. Many people find that they learn more about intimacy (that is, themselves) by being parents than in any other way. We do not choose our children, yet their genetic blueprint, containing as it does elements from both ourselves and our partner, forces us to confront deep issues in our own blueprint and its expression in daily life. The wise individual grows hugely from his or her parenting experiences and, with luck and care, some of the fruits of this learning are passed on to the next generation. It can also benefit the parents' relationship, though most couples do not get the best they could out of such lessons. To be fair, few of us gain as much as we could from most of life's lessons.

WHAT IS INTIMATE BEHAVIOUR?

We have looked at the style and nature of intimate relationships between lovers, but how can we tell that two people are *behaving* in an intimate way? Definitions of what seems truly intimate vary hugely and many a good partnership falters because of this. It is therefore useful to look now at some of the things that intimates do together.

TALKING

This always comes high on the list but, as we shall see on page 129, listening is probably more important. Talking can certainly enable us to reveal ourselves, but much communication takes place between intimates on a non-verbal plane. We do not have to be forever talking in order to be intimate. In fact many couples talk too much, using it unconsciously as a defence against doing other, more important, business together.

Most of us find a private moment such as this very touching. Accepting a gift directly into our mouth is an activity we reserve for those with whom we are exceptionally intimate.

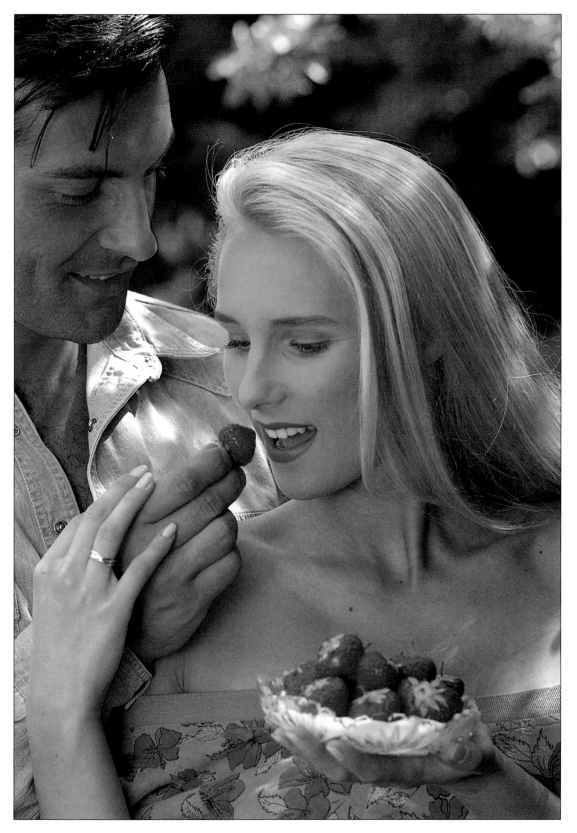

SILENCE

In the complex web of intimate communication, silence has its part to play too. Comfortable intimates use it a lot. To new couples just starting out on their journey of discovery, however, silence can seem somewhat threatening and many avoid it. This is hardly surprising in a culture that is unused to silence.

LAUGHING AND CRYING TOGETHER

These are greatly undervalued as sources of intimacy. Many couples I see rarely laugh together and hardly ever cry in one another's presence. Given that both are important ways of dealing with deep issues in our heart and soul, this is a great loss. Sometimes crying or laughing is far from intimate, however, such as laughing *at* our partner or crying because he or she has been foul to us. What I am referring to is the intimate sharing of deep joys and pains with our special person in a way that would be unlikely with anyone else. I have found that most men do not cry easily in the presence of their lover. They will often cry more readily with me alone but see it as weakness rather than an opportunity for increased intimacy to do so with their lover. Some of the best accolades I receive are from women who tell me how greatly improved their intimate life is now that their husband can cry in their presence.

TOUCHING AND BEING TOUCHED

Physical touch is seen as the ultimate expression of intimacy in our society. Many couples, however, do not touch each other intimately apart from when they are having sex. For such couples, experiencing touch other than during foreplay or sexual intercourse can be hugely rewarding, even magical. I find it fascinating that of the thirty-five books I have written so far, my second-biggest seller is a book about massage. My number-one seller is about non-intercourse sex. Clearly there is a considerable interest in non-genital physical activity between men and women. My clinical experience tells me that this interest is increasing healthily as couples think again about genital sex being the ultimate in human connection and as AIDS makes genital business more hazardous for those at risk.

Often the touching of bodies leads to a touching of minds or souls. I was working with a woman recently who started to sob when I tucked her up in a blanket as she lay on a mattress. Through her tears she moaned that it was about the nicest thing anyone had done for her in years. She proceeded to get in touch with the previously unacknowledged pain of having a partner who only ever touched her when he wanted sex.

TENDERNESS

This commodity is often in short supply in many so-called intimate relationships, yet I believe that we cannot truly say we are intimate if we are not tender with our lover. The graciousness that goes with tenderness somehow ennobles both the giver and the receiver. Such love is at the heart of courtly behaviour and enhances our intimate life. Tenderness also spreads to other areas of our life and enables us to be more gracious there too.

TRUST

This is perhaps one of the emotions that people mention most often when dis-cussing intimacy. Given that the intimate life calls for considerable bravery as we start to be really ourselves in the presence of another, it is unlikely that we will go far if that person is untrustworthy. Millions of people find it hard to trust *anyone*, not just their partner. The root of this problem lies in the way in which so many babies are reared. Males in our culture are brought up to be self-sufficient and not to trust people until they are sure of them or find themselves in a situation in which they have no choice but to do so.

HONESTY AND OPENNESS

No intimate relationship can flourish without these two commodities. This does not mean that we have to tell all our secrets, especially from the past. People often ask me whether they should 'come clean' with their partner about something that happened long ago on the basis that 'this is how I really am/was and in an intimate relationship my lover should know all about this real me'. I find this fallacious and even dangerous. Most people do not want or need to have a blow-by-blow account of the things in life that shaped their partner. Although this *can* sometimes be help-ful, it should only be done in response to a very specific event or occasion. Getting out the dirty washing from years ago rarely helps. After all, when we take on our loved one we do not do so on a money-back guarantee basis. Intimate lovers have enough trust to take as they find and love each other *because* of their pasts. No matter what the past contains, it has created the unique individual they love.

FORGIVENESS

None of us can hope to live together without creating some hurt for our partner from time to time. And where there is hurt, forgiveness will be called for, yet this subject is little talked about these days. We look at it in more depth on page 85.

DISCIPLINE

This is a rather unfashionable word today with its connotations of 'being told off'. However, we all need to be *self*-disciplined. A lot of the bad behaviour I see between couples stems from poor discipline and many who say they want to explore intimacy are too undisciplined to make any helpful changes. Creating a more intimate life calls for more effort, at least early on. Once the system works on autopilot much less daily input is required.

It is often said that we have to work at a relationship if it is to succeed. I find this a rather unappealing concept. Most of us work hard enough to cope with our jobs, families, travel, money worries, housing problems and so on. The thought of adding yet another burden is highly unattractive to many. Creating a more intimate life does not call for work in the commonly used sense of the word, but it does demand more discipline, energy and effort, much of which can be so rewarding that it should really be thought of as recreation, or rather re-creation. Many individ-uals 'work' far harder at their hobbies and leisure activities than they do at their relationships.

COMMITMENT

None of the above points will mean much unless we are capable of commitment to our special relationship. This makes us feel that all our efforts and energy are worth investing. I use the word 'investing' because, although we cannot be sure of what the return will be or even what form it will take, most couples who travel the road to increased intimacy do find that they reap a dividend from their efforts. Few of us, though, will make such an investment without some sort of commitment that guarantees our efforts will not be in vain. In reality, any progress we make towards intimacy stands us in good stead for all future relationships as the real work we do is on ourselves. For more on this subject, see page 42.

IS THE PURSUIT OF INTIMACY WOMEN'S WORK?

Women are generally considered to be more able at emotional matters, and looking after relationships is seen as women's work. This has certainly been the case historically and is still true in millions of relationships around the Western world. This does not mean that women need relationships more than men do. In fact, quite the contrary is true, as we shall see on page 76. It appears that men have mainly been involved in other matters and have left the responsibility for emotional and relationship issues to females. Even today, men still find it more difficult and less immediately rewarding to improve their personal and emotional skills, unless it helps them in other more obviously masculine ways, such as at work.

Much of this dates back to the relatively subordinate position of women in largely male-dominated Western cultures. In any relationship between two groups of unequal status, the 'lower' group always seeks to understand the 'superior' one, rather than vice versa. Blacks and various immigrant minorities, for example, know much more about white rules and cultural roles than the other way around. So it was that females were reared to hone their relationship skills to attract and keep a man and then to look after a family.

Although there is much debate as to whether females have innate caring and relational abilities that men lack, the argument is probably sterile in today's world. Whatever the biology of the situation, social changes have made it imperative that men alter their attitudes and behaviour to share in the work of relationship creation and maintenance. We shall see how men fare with this on page 67.

I have little doubt that men will see no need to change as long as their women and females in general disable them on this matter. Even today, many women still seek to please and appease men in an unhealthy way; many bend over backwards to conform to male-dominated cultural norms when these are clearly unhelpful to both sexes; many retain and maintain their power over men by appropriating emotional issues within relationships; and many give men the impression that to be interested in emotional and relationship issues is second-class work, that is, looked at historically, women's work.

The woman is her own worst enemy in many of the couples I see. She almost apologizes for her interest in emotional and relationship issues and then paradoxically wonders why it is that her man sees the whole thing as too unimportant for *him* to spend time on. Many women say something like, 'I expect I'm just too fussy/demanding/bullying/neurotic', when I talk this through with them. A man in a relationship with such a woman agrees with her and is confirmed in his/her view that it is all rather a waste of time and best left to 'silly women'.

Even some women who are positive and assertive about their skills in this area find themselves protecting their man from taking equal responsibility for intimacy issues in the relationship. This is not only unfair, leading to bitterness, frustration and disappointment in many women, sometimes for a whole lifetime, but also ensures that men will never improve.

The training for all of this starts early in life. Mothers expect less from their boys in this area than from their girls, and children expect less from their father than from their mother. As long as females take on the sole responsibility for relationship issues, men will never change. Men *are* changing slowly in these matters though, as I point out in the section starting on page 67. Perhaps in fifty years' time, as males of all ages are rewarded for their efforts at 'being' instead of just 'doing', things *will* change for the better. I see signs of improvement in younger couples and also in elderly ones, so perhaps significant change is not too far away in evolutionary terms.

INTIMACY AROUND THE WORLD

Most of us tend to think that intimacy is experienced in the same way by people the world over, yet this is almost certainly not so. There is much to be learned about international expectations of intimacy by first examining the way in which a society is constructed and how people are encouraged to behave within it.

Numerous studies have found that different countries value different relationship patterns. For example, individualistic cultures such as the USA emphasize individual rights, wants and goals whereas collectivist cultures such as Japan put stress on mutual obligation, needs and interdependency. People in American-type cultures tend to communicate directly with each other in an explicit way whereas the Japanese model produces results through more implicit means of communication.

Collectivist societies have many group systems – extended family, work-groups or neighbours – in which people have somewhat diffuse mutual obligations based on set status patterns. Such societies value conformity, tradition and behaviour patterns that benefit the group as opposed to the individual. In contrast, people within individualistic societies verbalize their needs more and are strongly self-assertive. One study found that the USA had a high individualism score, France a medium one and Japan a relatively low one.

Romance and one-to-one intimacy are, generally speaking, rated low in countries where family and group ties are important and high where they are not. As a result, individualistic cultures tend to put high values on one-to-one relationships, with all their stresses and anxieties, whilst collectivist cultures play this down, expressing personal love and intimacy more discreetly and implicitly.

French culture provides an interesting blend of the two models, combining, as it does, values of individuality and collectivism. For many Americans, individualism implies non-conformity whilst 'expressing oneself' means doing something just

Continued on page 20

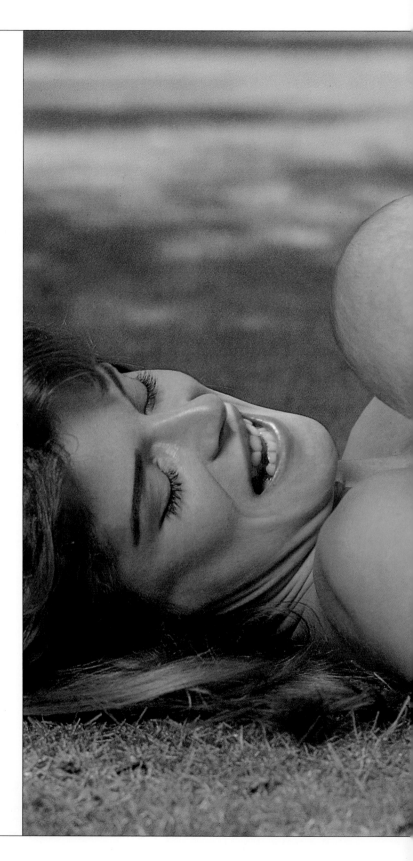

Most of us have our first experience of delicious intimate connection with another when we are babies. This is our early training ground. Lessons learned here can set us up for life. Those who do not have such opportunities, however, miss out and can find it difficult, or even impossible, to make up the loss in later life.

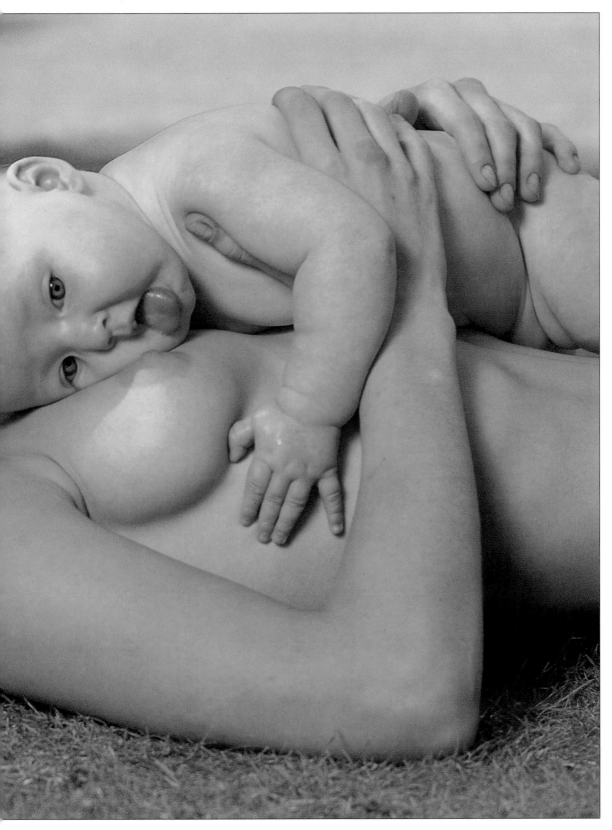

that bit differently from the next man. The French, however, see no problem with combining the two. This enables them to be true individualists yet also to experience and express this in the context of socially cohesive networks.

Masculine cultures, such as Japan and the USA, also favour clear definitions of gender roles, with males being assertive and females nurturing. Feminine cultures such as France, however, have much more fluid gender boundaries. Although males and females express intimacy differently in masculine cultures, they do not differ much in France. Could this be why Frenchmen are renowned as great lovers?

CHILDHOOD ORIGINS OF INTIMACY

If we are to understand why intimacy is such a vexed issue for so many adults we need to start by looking at how children are reared in Western society. Our upbringing has fateful effects on the rest of our lives and how we conduct our adult relationships.

Although I am not a child psychologist I have learned hugely from regression work that I regularly carry out with my patients. These insights provide windows on the past, even as far back as the womb itself, as people relive experiences that are inaccessible to their conscious mind. This is, however, a complex area about which no one can know the truth. We are all exploring and trying to find a way.

Starting at the beginning, therefore, it seems reasonable to assume that the foetus itself feels somewhat 'intimate' within its mother's womb. Although we have no direct way of knowing what unborn babies feel, modern research is starting to substantiate what pregnant women have been saying for centuries: that a baby's emotions and behaviour can be affected by its mother's own experiences. To me, this seems to be beyond doubt. So perhaps our very first experience of feeling safe, 'loved', wanted and valued, occurs in the womb. There is now a significant body of research that shows that the birth process itself can also modify an individual's personality. Clearly a great deal has already happened at the experiential and emotional level before a new-born baby first finds itself in its mother's arms.

Once born, human babies are exceptionally dependent and vulnerable compared with the young of other animal species. A baby cannot care for itself and is totally at the mercy of the adults around it if it is to be fed, cleaned, clothed, sheltered and loved. This makes it very vulnerable to the attention of its significant adults, a vulnerability that persists throughout our lives in one form or another.

In our culture, and indeed in most around the world, it is women who do most of the caring for babies and very young children. This 'mothering' is probably the most basic influence on our lives and affects the whole of our relationships with others, especially those with whom we pair-bond in later life. So when we use the word 'mother' we think consciously and unconsciously of our own, real mother and also of women in general who behave in ways that are congruent with our model of mothering.

As babies we do not come to our innermost images of mothers just by *direct* experience of our mother; we also unconsciously construct other models in a complex way. We start to create an inner world consisting of 'objects' that are not so much real as personal representations of reality. So it is that a baby made to wait for a long time for the breast or bottle becomes angry and frustrated and, being too young to understand that the food-supplying object is something to do with its mother, comes to hate the breast or bottle itself for letting him down. The child now internalizes an image of the 'bad breast/bottle', which is real to him and this becomes part of his unconscious data bank. A baby who has such an internalized model can now deal with the 'bad breast/bottle' separately from its mother and so preserve its love for her whilst hating the 'naughty breast/bottle'. This is probably a way in which human infants come to terms with the real frustrations and pains of being so dependent. To hate one's actual mother might, the baby reasons, drive her away and then he really would die from lack of care. Having some sort of symbolic hate object is clearly a lot safer than hating the mother herself.

As a baby grows and becomes aware that the breast or bottle is part of or an extension of the real mother and not simply a source of life-giving milk in itself, he starts to build a more complete picture of what his mother is. As he grows older he builds layer after layer on to his experience of 'mothering'. By the time he goes to school his definition of a 'mother' is very different from what it was in the first few weeks after birth. However, as regression work shows, nothing we experience is ever forgotten. It simply sits in our unconscious data bank waiting to be accessed in response to some sort of trigger later in life.

Within the whole of this process we have to learn where the boundaries are between us and our mother. At first, in the womb, it must be very difficult for a baby to know how separate it is from its mother. At that time it could justifiably be claimed that the foetus is hardly separate at all, given that it relies entirely on its mother for its existence. It also mirrors *her* feelings, as any pregnant woman can attest. After birth, for those first nine months of 'pregnancy outside the womb' a baby is still totally dependent yet must now be able to make at least some observations as to the differences between itself and its mother.

As we have seen, being attached to our mother is vital for life itself in the earliest months of life. It is hardly surprising then that any threat to this attachment brings the huge anxiety that we might be left to die. Just how much our mother does for us on an unconditionally loving basis will largely determine how safe we feel in this insecure world when we can do so little for ourselves.

In order that babies will be cared for, nature has designed them to be attractive and appealing. A mother can also obtain satisfaction from her efforts at caring and nurturing, often way beyond what she ever thought likely before she was pregnant. But there is always tension between the mother's need to be independent to lead her own life – and her baby's undeniable need to be totally cared for day and night. This leads to all kinds of 'battles' between the two with both craving separation and togetherness at a primitive, unconscious level. The mother also resonates with her inner fears of abandonment from her own days as a helpless baby. The fears, thrills, delights, horrors and anxieties of separation and unity are deeply embedded in our unconscious, ready to emerge as continuing themes in adult life.

Whenever, as adults, we find ourselves in a one-to-one relationship that matters to us, we experience again those early struggles between separation and unity. We relive the delights of going off as a toddler to explore the world, hoping and trust-

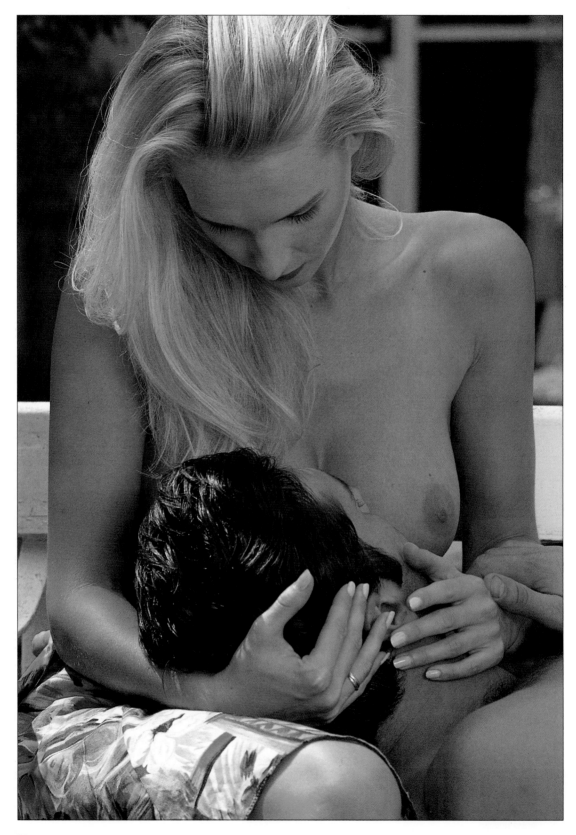

ing that our mother will be there, even if we temporarily lose sight of her. We repeatedly re-experience the pleasures of being reunited with our mother after any sort of separation. This is the bedrock of the agony and ecstasy of any symbiotic, one-to-one union. Ecstasy, because in our mother's womb and later in her arms we knew the bliss of being safe, wanted, loved and warm. Agony, because from the moment of cutting the umbilical cord life is all about separations, each one experienced as at least a symbolic threat to survival itself.

At the conscious level we know as adults that we cannot possibly return to that old symbiotic union. The little child within us yearns for it, however, and our adult self behaves as if those ancient feelings and experiences were not very far from consciousness. So it is that we long for connection with another, only to feel somewhat uncomfortable when we get it and anxious lest it be taken away.

The way we bring up children in the West today is often unhelpful in this context. For at least a century now it has been supposed that babies should be parted from their mothers as early as possible to make them more independent. Wet-nursing in the last century, nannies and, in later life, boarding schools are manifestations of enforced separation 'for the sake of the children'.

Everything I know from my work with 'adult children', however, tells me that no child can be forcibly separated from his mother without considerable problems later in life. There is only one way to create independent children and that is to allow them to be healthily dependent for as long as they need. Then, from this position of safety and self-confidence, they can go out into the world and claim their independence. Such an individual can eventually find another who is like-minded and make a life together that is based on *inter*dependence.

Children cannot hope to separate healthily from their mothers and have any sense of self itself unless they first learn about the core of themselves: the self within. Only when this coherent, independent sense of self, which makes us uniquely different from others, has been incorporated can we function in the world and have our primary needs met. This struggle to know the self within is parallel but different for boys and girls because they are both being mothered by a female. It is soon obvious to a boy that being male is different from being female but what is not so easy is working out what these differences signify outside the simple anatomical variations.

An early task for a boy is to renounce his connection with his mother so that he can start to identify with his maleness and so manifest his difference from her. His father will, until now, have been a somewhat shadowy figure and may, in modern society, even be largely absent. It has been calculated that approximately four out of ten families in the USA, for example, have no adult male living with them. Millions of men work such long hours away from home that their wives are effectively

---

Many men find that this sort of regression to babyhood helps them relive the joys of those times. Others, for whom such unconditional acceptance was rare in their early years, may use the opportunity to experience baby-like intimacy and so heal their old wounds.

single parents. Not every boy is brought up in such a home and most have the opportunity to forge some sort of relationship with their father. At around the age of seven they start empathically to enter the world of men.

To protect himself from the pain of the separation from his mother the little boy builds up a set of unconscious defences that he will carry for the rest of his life. He now adds these to his existing boundary concepts that differentiate him from his mother as a biological being and starts to see himself as separate and different from her. Adult males can call up such defences when their one-to-one relationship is threatened or threatening. Indeed, it appears that some 'grown-up little boys' never really come to terms with having been abandoned by their mother. This in itself leads to a distrust of her, and, by implication, all females. I see many who harbour great hatred and distrust of females in general. At first they are loath to accept that this might have started all those years ago, but with regression therapy they soon experience, or rather re-experience, the reality of it. Such feelings take their toll in the bedrooms of such adult boys as they look out for betrayal at the hands of yet another woman whom they love and are trying to trust.

Girls have quite another set of tasks to achieve in early life. As they are physically somewhat like their mothers they do not have to break away in order to accept and define their biological difference. Similarly there is no need to build up defences against feeling and attachment and thus less need for the rigid boundaries that males develop to protect and maintain their defences. A female's 'self' definition is thus more fluid than a male's. But because she has not had to separate herself so completely from her mother, she has other work to do if she is to be sure that she is in fact *not* her mother. A part of this entails being aware of what her mother is thinking and feeling. Additionally, the girl has both mother and father, and their relationship to deal with, unlike the boy who largely comes to identify with his father only. The girl thus has three people in a triangle, while the boy has two in a line: his father and himself. All of this seems to make little girls more aware of their own feelings and those of others and is said to be the reason they become more skilled at empathy.

But girls have other problems with their mothers. There is, in fact, increasing concern about children being brought up only by women. The role and importance of fathering is now better understood and its absence is being linked to difficulties in forming intimate bonds.

The girl within the adult woman has come from a somewhat non-erotic relationship with her mother in the earliest formative years so as an adult she seeks a brighter-coloured world of love. She therefore seeks a man who will restore her inner unity, which was damaged when her mother set her up as a 'loved object' (which she was) and a 'desired subject' (which she was not). When we are an 'object', in psychological jargon, we become what another significant person thinks we are or needs us to be (even if it is only in this person's eyes). A 'subject' in this sense is what we think or feel we are. I see many women who have difficulty in unifying the 'sex object who can be desired' with the 'subject who can be valued' so that they can feel like a whole person. Many a woman's grasping for a man stems from this need to be a good enough 'object' for someone.

Many women find it difficult to believe that they are a 'good enough object', even when repeatedly told so by their lover. This forces them repeatedly to ask 'Do you *really* love me?' and to look constantly for reassurance through clothes, make-up and, at a more extreme level, plastic surgery. Her man, however, sees this cry for reassurance for the anxiety it is, and her demands as a sign that he is about to be possessed or devoured. This then triggers old memories of having to get away from his mother to be 'separate' and 'different'. Trouble brews. She, feeling unloved and unmothered, may seek solace in her own children or become 'mentally ill' or 'depressed' so that she can compel a doctor or therapist to become the 'good mother' she never had and her husband refuses to be.

All of this is further complicated by the playing out of unresolved Oedipal issues that lurk in all of us to some degree. Almost every parent is aware of his or her opposite-sex child's love for them at around three to five years of age. Little boys say that they will marry their Mummy and girls that they wish Mummy would go away and let them have Daddy to themselves. This normal phase of child psychosexual development is healthy in that we come to focus on the opposite-sex parent as a safe 'love object'. The only danger is if the child actually obtains this love object in reality instead of in fantasy. This is one reason child sexual abuse is so harmful.

The essence of all Oedipal connections at this age is that they must not be actualized. As long as the yearning for the idealized opposite-sex parent remains only in the fantasy world of the young child, he or she will have sufficient drive to go out one day in later life and find a love object with whom to bond. I see many adults who in some real way obtained their opposite-sex parent (though not necessarily genitally) when they were children. This stifles their ability to create relationships with the opposite sex later in life and wreaks havoc in their sexual lives. Such 'spiritual incest', as I call it, can be as devastating as real incest in that it disables the child and damages them hugely. Almost always, of course, it is the parent who is at fault in that he or she is acting out his or her own unmet unconscious needs, using the child as an innocent party to achieve this. So it is that some girls are 'little wives' to their dads and boys 'little men' to their mothers. So strong is the tie to such models that man-woman relationships later are doomed to failure until all this is worked out and worked through consciously.

Some of this will ring bells with many readers, and it is easy to see how it could be a barrier to intimacy. So it is that we all unconsciously try to re-create situations in which we can rework unsatisfactory and unsatisfied material from our long-lost pasts within our current relationship. A man, for example, may become very jealous of his new baby. It is not that he does not want to be a father; dislikes babies in general; or does not want family life (though any or all of these might be the case). Rather he is unconsciously acting out his unremembered but painful past as he experiences the new baby as something the wife has created to marginalize him and even abandon him as his mother did, or threatened to do, all those years ago. His unconscious hatred of her for doing this can be projected on to the new baby or on to his wife; or, more subtly and perversely, can be expressed as extreme demonstrations of love for either or both as his unconscious battles to cover up the ancient hatred and fear.

Continued on page 28

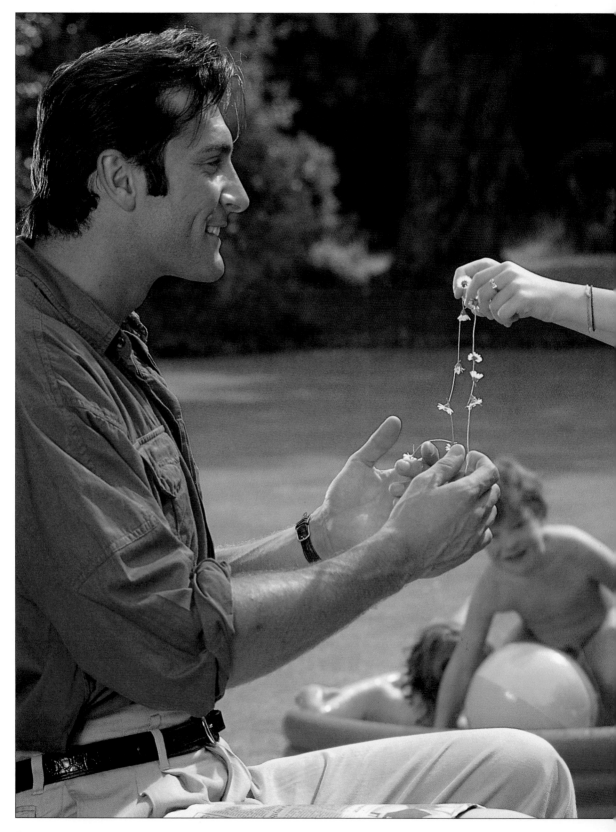

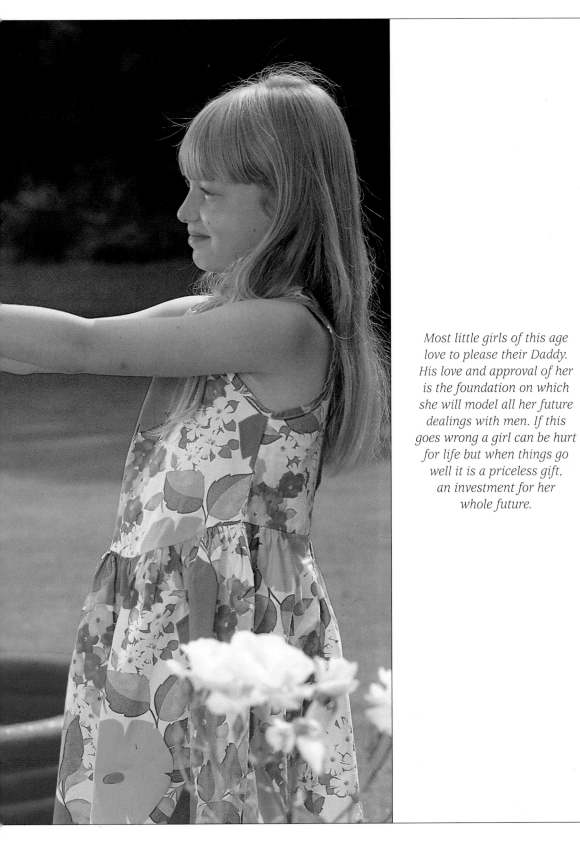

*Most little girls of this age
love to please their Daddy.
His love and approval of her
is the foundation on which
she will model all her future
dealings with men. If this
goes wrong a girl can be hurt
for life but when things go
well it is a priceless gift,
an investment for her
whole future.*

Men in general have problems forming an exclusive relationship with a female because they are terrified by the ambivalence intrinsic to the attachment this involves. This oscillation between emotional connection and his fear of it makes him a difficult partner with whom to be intimate. It also creates friction between the pair as he seeks to re-create the 'perfect mother' scenario and she tries to make up for the deficiencies of *her* childhood.

There is no doubt that mothers behave and feel differently towards male and female children. Most girls, as non-Oedipal objects for their mother, know that they are unsatisfying and unsatisfactory. The girl, and later the woman, is never wholly satisfied with what she is or how she looks. All women want to change something about themselves and particularly their bodies. My research into this showed that three-quarters of the 300 women I questioned were dissatisfied with their bodies in one way or another. This, I believe, originates from the time when it was all too plain to the little girl that she did not excite the level of interest and desire in her mother that her brothers did. In this sense a little girl starts to deny her sexuality because, she is taught, it is something that she will experience later as a woman with a man. Boys are accepted simply because they are male whereas girls have continually to prove that they are feminine. So it is that 'being like mother', an identification, takes precedence over 'being oneself', which is valid in itself. Ironically, the little girl is not even like her mother physically. She has no breasts, pubic hair, periods or babies. Yet she is not like her father either. She cannot, therefore, identify with her mother in any deep way and same-sex feelings between them are out of bounds. I have heard many mothers tell of how they kiss their little boy's penis as they wash and dry him but I have never heard mothers recounting parallel tales of female-to-female business. It is not until adolescence that a girl realizes that there are other bodies like hers. I have yet to meet a woman who talks to her little daughter about the clitoris yet the penis is openly acknowledged in millions of mother-son interactions.

So because she has no sex and no sexual object (her father is usually absent) the little girl starts to repress her sexuality. This, I believe, is just the beginning of women's distrust of one another, a situation that persists for many throughout their whole lives. Many's the woman who has told me that it is females, not males, who are her worst enemies at work or play. This distrust is probably the basis for female empathy as girls learn very young how to read their mother's emotions and so keep on the good side of her. Girls are much more watchful and vigilant of the emotions of others than are boys but this might not be as healthy as at first appears (see also page 77).

From this situation in which mothers do almost all child-rearing, especially of the malleable, young pre-schooler, we all emerge somewhat damaged. In men it can take the form of a resentment of women, which all men suffer to some degree. Most never recover. In a woman it is seen as a mad search for male approval in a world where she 'knows' she cannot trust women. Her very existence revolves around creating and sustaining connection with a man to make up for the poverty of connection she had with her mother. Her desperate 'need' for a man to repair her earlier losses and longings for the father she did not have in early childhood makes her man feel trapped as it becomes clear at the unconscious level that he is going to have to fill many roles. She is now set up for jealousy of other women and he for a hatred and fear of women who seek to control and trap him by their emotional neediness.

Is it difficult, given this background, to see how intimacy fails to develop? If we are to alter any of this, fundamental changes will have to be made in the way we bring up children. At the moment, our drive for material wealth forces fathers out of the home and to be largely absent. Whilst gaining material comfort, however, we create psychic problems as women are left exclusively to bring up children. Divorce also plays its part, with millions of youngsters having no male in their home. This creates a somewhat new scenario in historical terms in that we have absent fathers and relatively over-present mothers, even if they work. Most mothers carry far too heavy a burden of parenting early in the life of their children and, as we have briefly explored, this has fateful effects for their children's ability to be intimate in later life.

Young babies and children need fathers *and* mothers or males and females at the very least if they are to avoid many of the pitfalls outlined in this chapter. If my assertions have any validity, we will have to review our thinking, attitudes and behaviour when it comes to parenting and child care in general. Most fathers see their parenting task as time-limited whereas almost all mothers see it as a lifetime's responsibility. By creating a situation in which mothers and other females have too great a responsibility for parenting we pay a terrible price in terms of adult relationships. If adult boys are to have more realistic views and experiences of women, surely they need to be parented by males who can then take some of the burden and responsibility for the blame that is currently aimed at females. This, of course, applies to all those who care for young children in day nurseries and other institutions for young children. As long as we keep men out of the creative processes involved in the psychic development of children we will build yet more divisions between the sexes and whole new generations of individuals who are incapable of being intimate.

Today's society is not geared to raising psychically balanced children. It makes few concessions to their needs. By doing so and by over-valuing mothering as opposed to dual-sex child care, we are erecting problems that can only replicate themselves. Perhaps the intimate couple with children can review all this and, as a result, rear offspring who are fundamentally capable of intimacy rather than having to graft it on later in life with all the attendant difficulties.

FEELINGS AND METAFEELINGS

However children are reared, emotions are at the root of all transactions between human beings, especially lovers. We cannot escape them. Emotions are the strong feelings that we all have from time to time, particularly in the company of those who mean most to us – our 'special' people. Some feelings are very obvious to ourselves and others; others are very difficult for an outsider to perceive; some are powerful, others very weak and so on. I list some of the more common emotions on page 132.

Almost every statement we make has at least some emotional content. The trouble is that often we do not realize what the emotion is or indeed that we are feeling anything at all. Our senses by and large give us fairly accurate feedback from the material world but our emotions often fool us, coming, as they do, largely from the unconscious recesses of our mind.

If Jill says, for example, 'I've got so much work to do before the meeting tomorrow', there are many emotions that could be hidden behind such an apparently simple remark. Is she *desperate* because she does not think she will get it all done? Does she *fear* that she might not be up to doing it at all? Is she really *asking* Peter to offer to cook the meal so that she can get on? And so on. Many interpretations are possible and even Jill herself may not know what it is that is making her feel the way she does. Does she even really know *what* she is feeling? It is possible she does not.

It is in this sort of situation that empathic listening comes into its own. Listening 'with a third ear' in this way allows us to put ourselves into our partner's shoes for a moment and really try to feel what he or she is feeling. All this is described in some detail on page 129. The end result is that our partner, troubled by his or her own emotions at that moment, finds understanding, company and support in the way that we feed back these emotions.

At first, this might seem somewhat wasteful of time and energy. 'After all', people ask me, 'If he's so angry, why doesn't he just get on with it and be angry? What have I got to do with it?' The thing to remember here is that as soon as we start to feel strongly about something life stops being simple for us. That particular emotion will have been experienced before by us and it is as though there is a button that has been pressed leading us into some sort of unconscious data bank of associated feelings and life events. The anger, or whatever, in the here-and-now, is no longer simply about the current issue. We start to live out old events and their attendant emotional states.

In the above incident, for example, perhaps Jill starts unconsciously to get in touch with her father's wrath at her leaving her homework until the last moment. She unconsciously remembers his response and automatically believes that Peter will behave in the same way that her father did. Suddenly the whole transaction becomes clouded by Jill's relationship with her father all those years ago and Peter is unwittingly drawn into it 'as if' he were her father. This understandably raises emotions in him that trigger off old memories from *his* past whether they involve Jill or not.

The only way around this sort of endless circuit of emotions is for the listener to reflect what he or she observes the other to be feeling. The speaker can then consciously realize what these feelings are; that another person can perceive them clearly; and that he or she is still wanted, loved and accepted even though the partner can see the effects the emotion is having.

We all crave to be accepted and understood when we are feeling strongly about something. It is so difficult for us to understand ourselves in these situations and we can so easily scare ourselves with our own powerful emotions that it feels healing to have our loved person stay with us and help us negotiate the stormy seas in which we find ourselves. Of course our partner cannot feel *for* us or do our emotional work for us, but simply by being he or she can give us the security we need to do the work ourselves. Often it feels far too dangerous and risky to do anything and we stay stuck with our emotions.

Learning how to become more empathic and tune into our partner's feelings can take a long time (see page 132). Most of us become quickly involved in our own business and take the focus off our partner who then feels that his or her emotions are unable to be dealt with by *anyone*. This can lead to a sense of desperation and, if persisted with for years, a real fear of going 'mad'.

Feelings, then, are an inevitable part of life. They are usually coped with in one of four ways: being empathically 'heard'; ignoring them; denying them; or projecting them on to others. Men, mainly because of their upbringing, usually seek to deny or ignore their feelings in various ways. By internalizing them, they store them away to be dealt with by other methods such as drinking, overwork, sex, or substance abuse. As boys they were taught to suppress feelings and their expression; as adults their fear of what might happen if they were not to do so paralyses them into inaction.

Whenever I run groups dealing with feelings most people raise various issues that are in reality nothing to do with feelings but rather to do with feelings *about* feelings. These have been called metafeelings. They are different from primary feelings. Primary feelings are things such as joy, anger, fear and rage: feelings we are born with the ability to express, or at least feel. Metafeelings are a less pure form of feeling because they arise out of our social conditioning. Examples are guilt, embarrassment, self-consciousness, hostility and shame. They are *learned* feelings and can be helpful or unhelpful to us. Clearly a sense of guilt can be useful socially, whereas if we say we feel 'tolerant' of our partner it makes us appear one up on him or her and as such does both of us harm.

In any journey towards greater intimacy we need to become more aware of what we are feeling at any time, what our partner is feeling and what the metafeelings are. By doing this we make ourselves more aware of what is *our* business and what is our partner's and can therefore allow our partner to be himself or herself while we are being ourselves.

A useful way of getting to grips with all this is to start listening to what people are saying as you go about your daily life at work or play. Try to name the main emotion that you perceive the parties are feeling. Observe their body language to obtain all the helpful information you can. Try to sort out the primary feelings from the feelings about feelings and see how both parties get themselves into trouble by mixing up all these things. Because you will be uninvolved, you will find it a useful training ground for your own relationship where, by definition, you will be less able to stand back and calmly take stock of the situation. After some months of practising this new level of perception on others, you should be able, with the help of the exercises in Part Three, to build your own skills in dealing with the feelings that involve you and your partner. Be prepared for all this to take some time because if, as is the case for most of us, you were brought up in a household where empathy was in short supply, you will find it difficult to change the habits of a lifetime.

LOVE, CLOSENESS AND INTIMACY

There can be few more confusing areas of man-woman relationships than the triangle represented by love, closeness and intimacy. Most people mix them up and find that striving for one often excludes experiencing the other two.

Trying to define love is well beyond a book of this scope. In broad terms every human interaction offers the possibility of love. But it is being loving that brings the benefits, not being loved. Showing love to another should be unconditional; without any expectation of being thought well of or obtaining sexual favours in return. Loving someone is a privilege not a chore.

All of this should be contrasted with being 'in love'. This sort of 'sickness' is a self-centred, often selfish state in which we make our partner into something that we consider valuable. It reflects *our* innermost needs and says little or nothing about our partner as a unique individual. By projecting our unconscious business from the past on to our beloved we try to force this person to be what we want. And this may bear little or no resemblance to whom he or she actually is.

This is not love. If I really love you it allows you to become fully you at that moment. This love encompasses both positive and negative traits. We know we are being loved when we experience being truly ourselves. And although it can be tricky sometimes to know if we are being *loving* it is not difficult to know when we feel *loved*.

It appears that we all need to love and to feel loved. Perhaps this is the way we can reassure ourselves that the loneliness and separation we fear (see page 21) will not claim us at that particular moment in life. Given that we all seem to need repeated reassurance that we are loved, the underlying wound, or fear of being wounded, must be very great or a one-shot immunization against it would suffice for life. But it does not.

Being 'in love' often precedes real love but it can make the latter more difficult. Many of us find we are so in love with the fantasy image of our partner, or even with love itself, that true love for our partner the way he or she really is can be impossible. Clearly, then, being 'in love' has little to do with intimacy. It usually falls away fairly quickly whilst intimacy is something that builds and endures as we continue to invest in one another.

Closeness is a commodity that many couples I see rate very highly. They believe that being together or close will bring them intimacy. On the vast majority of occasions, however, they are disappointed. Paradoxically, closeness, or perhaps more accurately, over-closeness, turns out to be the enemy of intimacy. The problem with being close is that when we are experiencing it we are more aware of our partner than we are of ourselves. Many couples are so fixed in their desire for closeness that they can never experience intimacy. They focus largely on one

Tender moments such as these give us the opportunity to enjoy love, closeness and intimacy. Relaxing in one another's company, just being ourselves, can be a real haven from the day-to-day pressures of life. Most of us can feel this safe only with our special person.

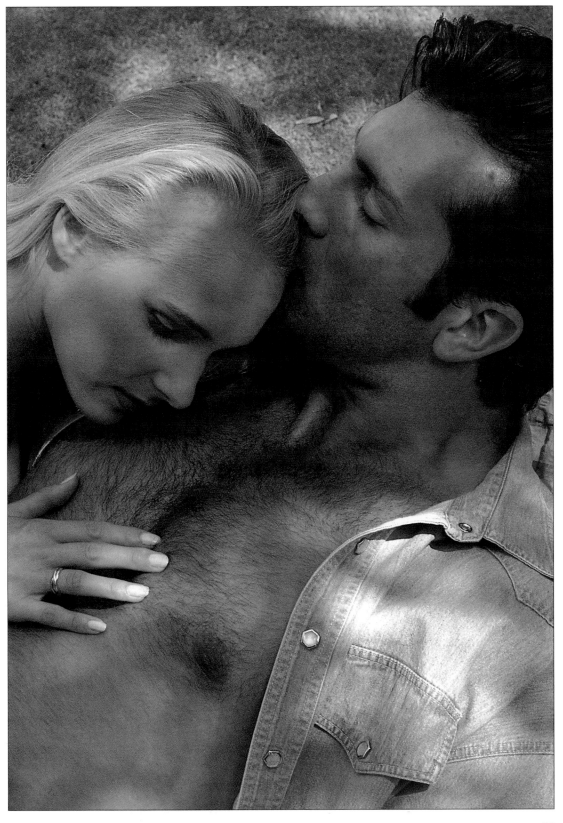

another and, if and when they can at last focus on themselves, they lose sight of their partner.

Of course it is possible to be healthily close. When we deal with someone we love we are indeed sensitive to his or her thoughts, feelings, needs, realities, unconscious and so on. This makes us somewhat more aware of this person's reality at that particular moment than we are of our own. However, many couples find that they very substantially focus on their partner's reality in a way that eclipses their own. This is not healthy closeness and precludes intimacy.

Healthy closeness is like a dance in which two people move well together, caring for and complementing one another. They are aware of one another's realities and can experience them as unique and special; and they are prepared to give up sectors of personal space to be selflessly loving, interested and caring. This reciprocal see-saw benefits both equally and makes intimacy more likely. None of this is like being unhealthily clinging or dependent on the other. If we are healthily close we willingly give up parts of ourselves to enable us to expand our awareness of our partner. If our partner is dependent on us we 'take care' of him or her. This is very different from 'caring'. The former is not possible within an intimate relationship but the latter is an integral part of one.

So being close enables us really to know *our beloved* and being intimate really to know *ourselves*. When we are close we know our *partner* in our presence; when we are intimate we know *ourselves* in our partner's presence. Most of us know ourselves only in our own personal space. Within an intimate relationship we can know ourselves in the presence of another. This makes us free, more alive, and able to grow.

Romantic love then has little to do with intimacy and closeness can be its enemy. These provocative thoughts are a good starting point for any couple seeking to build a more intimate life together. Ask yourselves how you think you love one another. Try to assess how unconditional your love for one another is. Thinking about the following questions may help you.

How clinging are you? Can you let your partner go? Does your love smother your partner? How do you cope with the see-saw that is an inevitable part of loving? Do you always want your see-saw to be static and in perfect balance? If so, where is the thrill and the motion in your loving life?

Does possessiveness get in the way of your love? Would you secretly like to own your partner? Do you look to your partner to supply all your unmet needs and wants in life? Do you believe that if your partner really loved you he or she would actually do this? How do you cope with misunderstandings? Do you feel that unless you are totally understood you are not really loved?

Do you believe that your partner should be a mind reader if he or she really loved you? Are you seduced by stereotypes that force a man to be 'strong' and woman 'weak' in the name of love? Do you expect your lover to take care of you? Do you harbour a secret wish to be cared for entirely and completely by your beloved? Is your relationship dogged by unconscious games that require rescuing/victimizing/punishing behaviour (see page 52)?

Do you find yourself wishing that things were how they used to be? Do you feel that love should conquer everything? Can your sort of love cope with change or does it live in the past, wishing the world and both of you would stay the way they were? Quite a provocative list, I think you will agree.

I hope that by talking through some of these questions you will be able to deal with love, closeness and intimacy more realistically within your relationship. We all have to find our own path through this maze and no book can do more than trigger some new thoughts that might slowly change attitudes.

Many of our abstract ideas of 'love' actually sabotage healthy closeness and intimacy. But unless we take time to talk through what all these concepts mean to us on a daily basis in our love lives we can spend a whole lifetime missing one another. Unfortunately, the vast majority of us have little or no training in any of this. Perhaps in some enlightened future, teenagers will be taught about such things at school so that as they start on the road of man-woman relationships they will have at least some sort of map to help them. I spend many hundreds of hours a year trying to help couples find their way on such a journey yet most are unaware that there even *is* a map. It is probably very difficult indeed to enjoy a fulfilling sex life in a lasting one-to-one relationship unless we can separate out love; closeness and intimacy. When we get it right, though, the rewards are formidable.

PAIRING WITH OUR SHADOW

There can be few people who work with relationships who do not quite quickly come to the conclusion that most couples choose one another on the basis of their deep, unconscious differences. At the superficial level, of course, we team up with someone who is overtly similar to us. This 'homogamy', as it is called, ensures that on an everyday basis we have enough similarity to be able to get along with one another. So it is that most of us form partnerships with someone who is of our approximate age, social class, education and intelligence level; someone from a somewhat similar geographical locality, of the same race, religion, with the same outlook on life, and so on.

At a much deeper level, however, we seem to seek out a mate who has (although we are not consciously aware of it at the time) a near-exact mirror of the dark side of our personality. This shadow side, a Jungian term for a concept that has been acknowledged since antiquity, is the part of our personality that we would rather not acknowledge or own; that we are afraid of; and that we most need to integrate within ourselves if we are to be whole. It is easy to accept the sunny side of our personality but much more difficult to look at the shadows within and own them as equal parts of ourselves, with their faults.

People who are very like us make good friends yet it is interesting that we rarely pair with them permanently. We seem to have affairs with those who are like us and marry those who are opposites. When we like someone similar to us we project our unconscious fantasies about ourselves on to the proposed mate and see the things we like about ourselves in this person. This is all very well for a short-term fling but somehow we know that this is not the path we should follow if we are to seek wholeness in our journey through life. For this we need a partner who is not simply a mirror of ourselves.

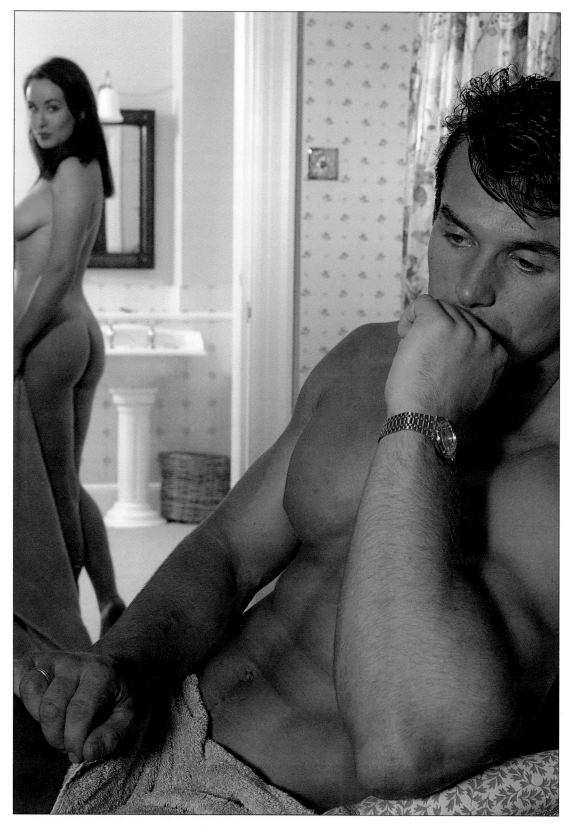

For this deeper business we crave someone who will enable us to battle against them for a whole lifetime because only by doing so do we stand a chance of struggling with our own inner devils and coming out healed. This sort of pairing clearly makes for a hard road but as countless couples have told me it is the only way that they can ever get anywhere as human beings. A working relationship calls for at least some work to be put into it.

Few of us can be married or live with someone for long before realizing that our partner thinks and behaves differently from ourselves. The trouble is that we all cherish the notion that we are normal and that the world is actually the way we see it. Living with someone as an intimate partner turns all this on its head as we struggle to accept that another person's way of looking at things might be right too.

Most of us see such differences as sources of conflict. This leads to trouble and damages intimacy. How about turning things round, though, and thinking of the different perceptions as sources of growth and knowledge instead? Now we can say with graciousness 'What are you seeing that I am not?'; 'What have you learned that I have yet to learn?'; or 'Could your way of looking at this issue actually be more appropriate than mine?' Intimate pair-bonding, usually in marriage in our culture, enables us constantly to play our 'reality' against that of another who loves us. The underlying love and care for one another, together with our sexual bond, can help us give and take in a way that benefits both.

When we make damning statements about our partner we are, if you think back to pairing with our shadow, actually often describing ourselves. 'You think only of yourself'; 'You're a mean bastard'; 'All you ever think about is sex'. Such statements are often really about our *own* unconscious shadow and many intuitive or wise people know this instinctively when they consult me about such issues in their marriage. Most of us can spot our partner's weak points a mile off; after all, according to what I am asserting here, that is why we chose this person. Unfortunately, many of us misuse this privileged information in a way that damages rather than enriches our partner.

As with all of our journey into intimacy the task is really to discover ourselves. Examining our criticisms of our partner can be a valuable way of gaining information about ourselves. It can also be extremely valuable to listen to what our partner has to say just in case he or she might be right, however much we would rather deny it. Denial is the very bedrock of trouble in this zone of partnership conflict. Whenever our beloved hits on a no-go area (see page 151) or reveals inner truths to us, we tend to go into denial mode. This reduces the pain in the here-and-now but actually harms us more in the long term because we shut ourselves out of an opportunity to learn and heal.

As long as we unconsciously choose someone who represents our psychological shadow there will be fights, disagreements and pain. Without such battles, however, we never grow. A couple in a good relationship can cope with the difficult emotional work involved in pairing with their shadow and turn it to their advantage.

There are several general principles around all this that seem to apply to many of the couples I see. The first is that if I am prepared to be open enough, some of my criticisms of my partner can help me pin-point and then own parts of my shadow self.

The second is that when I repeatedly criticize or make sweeping statements about my partner I am simply describing a part of myself I cannot readily own. I often see this in my sexual work with a couple. When one attacks the other for 'always wanting sex' I know that we are not far away from that individual confronting their inner and unconscious desire to show more interest in the subject. After some weeks in therapy this becomes an issue on which we can all have a laugh, so obvious does it become.

Thirdly, most of my partner's criticisms of me have at least some basis in reality. Given that my perception of reality is so imperfect and so biased towards me and my partial view of the world, I should consider it an honour that my partner criticizes me (provided he or she is not aggressive or hostile) because there are so few people who would care enough about whether I healed myself or not.

Lastly, many of the repeated, unthinking, emotional criticisms that I have of my partner reflect many of my unmet needs. I might, for example, scream at my partner that she is unbearably untidy whereas underneath I might be just as untidy, even if it is not readily obvious to the outside world. What, for example, have I done to counteract this inner dread of untidiness in myself? What negative effects might this sort of defence against my untidiness have had on our relationship?

How about asking the question, 'Is what I'm criticizing in my partner true of me too?' If we start to think constructively like this instead of projecting our own dirty laundry on to our partner so that by disowning him or her we can disown *it*, things really start to improve and intimacy flourishes.

All of this clearly calls for considerable humility and openness as we battle with our inner pains, unmet needs, ancient hurts, unfinished business from our original family, and so on. Yet in an intimate relationship this sort of battling becomes a route to greater insight. This in turn translates into more acceptance, graciousness and tolerance. And these commodities are at the very heart of an intimate relationship. Sex in such a union flourishes quite naturally as both partners see themselves growing and healing day by day.

LIKING ONE ANOTHER

'Liking' our partner sounds a rather shallow reason for living together. 'Love' sounds much more lofty, romantic and worth while. Yet simply liking a lover is greatly underestimated by most people. This is partly because it seems too uncomplicated to be of value.

When we choose a partner we do so largely on the basis of looks and personality. Other matters are later taken into account as the relationship deepens. Very often people who appear suited at the initial, superficial levels do not like one another very much. So such a woman can truly say 'I love Jim' yet be unaware of the reality, which is that she does not actually *like* him. Most of us would claim to try to 'love' humankind in general but few would claim to like everyone we meet.

I believe that intimacy can develop and grow only if the people involved like one another. I am not nearly as concerned about whether they 'love' one another in the commonly used sense of the word and I am not at all concerned about whether they are 'in love' with each other. Protestations of love or being in love tend to be genuine at the time but fade with experience. A real liking for someone is a far more solid basis for intimacy.

What makes us like someone is difficult to define. Being 'like' them is a good start; as is being liked by them. But neither of these is indispensable as we can like people who are very different from us and even those who do not like us. Usually we tend to like those who show us the side of ourselves we like to see. While this is not a sufficient basis in itself for an intimate relationship, it can be a good start. And perhaps the somewhat carefree nature of liking can create the leisurely background we need if we are to start on our journey towards intimacy. Those who like one another find, just as dancing couples do, that they move as one to create a system of togetherness and space that is mutually rewarding.

Liking means that we value our relationship more than we do our personal differences. This in turn means that we can hold very different positions and yet remain friends. We look at accepting difference on page 133. Such a couple knows when to be quiet rather than press an issue to prove themselves 'right' and will do deals with themselves and their partner rather than jeopardize the relationship. Many an atrocity has been committed in the name of love and couples who are 'in love' can hurt one another terribly. Those who genuinely like each other, however, do not sink to such lows.

If we really like one another we can afford to be flexible. This in turn allows us to cope with the uncertainties that are inherent in any relationship between human beings, not just between lovers. The old battle between wanting to be together and wanting to be alone rages year after year in most of us until we experience deep intimacy with ourselves and our partner. For most of us, then, liking our partner is an essential way of remaining flexible enough to make this journey with any safety.

As we age together as a couple liking usually deepens. The dance of life becomes more congenial and expectations more realistic. People often ask me why it is that elderly couples on television dating shows always seem to get on better than younger ones. What I perceive when I watch such programmes is that the older people *like* one another more than do the youngsters. Perhaps their longer experience of life has taught them how to like people more readily.

When working with troubled couples I often find that dislike is never far away. Personal habits are criticized, appearance endlessly faulted and behaviour damned. Rather than condemn the whole personality, as most such people do, I suggest that they look at the individual behind the behaviour: the person they once loved and cherished as a valued partner. Once we separate the individual from his or her behaviour things start to improve and we begin to like one another again.

But perhaps one of the greatest benefits that comes from liking one another is that it permits us to change. Liking is not pushy or demanding. Neither is it conditional, as many people claim their love for one another is. It is altogether more low-key and accepting and this is vital if we are to be free to change. Wherever we

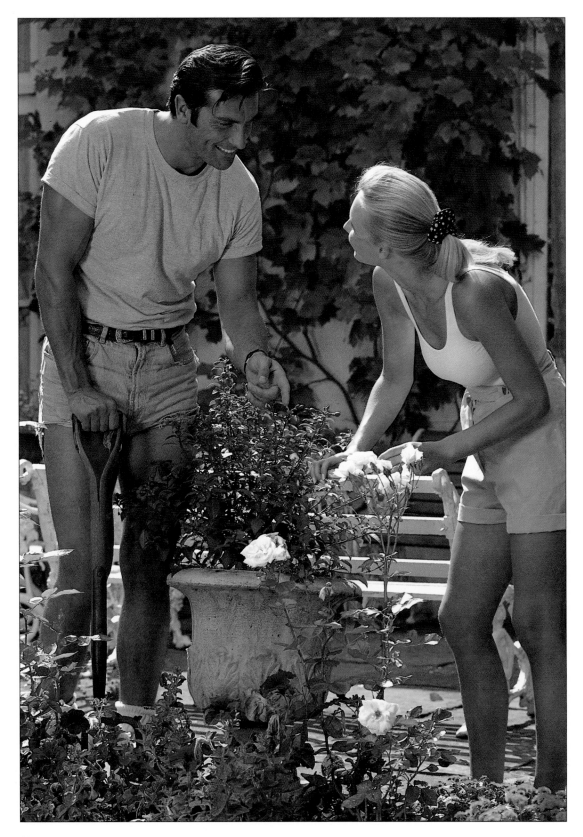

start in our lives together we are bound to change. Adjusting to this change is hard for most of us. Much of the difficulty arises because we are working on shifting sands the whole time. Just when we think we know what we want to change and have worked out a way to do so, situations in life generally or in our relationship in particular alter, throwing our plans into confusion. To make matters even more complicated, the world outside our relationship is also changing. This makes deciding who is 'right' on any issue almost impossible because today's attitudes and beliefs can be rendered redundant in a remarkably short time. This is probably more true today than ever before in history. Many young people cherish the notion that they will be able to change their partner in some way to make them more acceptable or 'right' for them. In my work as an 'Agony Uncle', this is the most common subject of letters from youngsters about to embark on marriage. It is a desire usually expressed more by women than men.

Perfection, however, is for the gods and our ideas of it, either in ourselves or in our partner, change quite quickly. Flawless companions exist only in the minds of flawed mates. No one with any personal integrity can possibly demand that their partner be more perfect than they themselves can be. People in therapy often say that they are only too well aware of their own failings but are not at all sure that they are able to put up with those of their partner! Do not forget when thinking about all this that our very method of choosing our partner ensures that we will be unhappy with them as imperfect models of humanity (see page 35) or we would not have got together in the first place. No one pairs with a clone of themselves because such a union would probably drive them mad. It is the management of the differences on a daily basis that makes life tricky for most of us. After all, no one is *always* late, sloppy, untidy, depressed, dependent, or whatever. Neither is anyone *always* happy, intimate, empathic, nurturing, and so on. We experience all of these things in our partner relative to our own position at the time and this position shifts from day to day let alone year to year.

Polarizing our partner's behaviour, then, does neither of us any favours and gets in the way of intimacy. Once we start to stereotype our lover – in or out of bed – we diminish the ability the person has to see himself or herself as bigger than a set of individual personality traits. We also limit our pleasure in our partner in this way. If we really like someone, even though we might not like all his or her behaviour, then we accept the person as he or she is and start on the long journey of liking ourselves. Do not forget that we have chosen our partner because he or she shows us our shadow side, and therefore what we so often dislike about our partner is really only a manifestation of the unconsciously unlikeable parts of ourselves. By practising liking our partner *because* of their 'faults' we allow ourselves to like our *self*. And, as we see throughout the book, this is the start of true intimacy.

Having fun and a shared life outside the bedroom is based on really liking one another. Just because we have great sex does not necessarily mean that we like one another yet liking is an essential basis for day-to-day demonstrations of intimacy.

DELIGHT, PLEASURE AND JOY

Many books about marriage and relationships in general are somewhat lightweight on the subjects of delight, pleasure and joy. It is as though the essence of a successful relationship is to work harder, try harder and get down to business. Whilst it is true that nothing much changes by wishful thinking alone it is also a fact that much progress occurs spontaneously when a couple delights in one another.

Couples today tend to spend so much time striving as parents, workers, employers, grandparents and so on that they rarely surrender themselves to pleasure. This is one reason why so many couples misuse sex by treating it as if it were the sole source of pleasure between them. For many this is indeed the case. Small wonder then that, in their relationship, so much hangs upon their sexual life.

I have outlined a helpful exercise on fun on page 155, but here let us look at a few ways that you might be able to inject some more delight, pleasure and joy into your sexual life. How about getting out of your usual routines, such as the time and place that you have sex? Try new positions, new locations and new times. Take more time for love-making, perhaps devoting a whole evening to 'making love' in the broadest sense before actual sexual intercourse. How about taking a short break away together, if only for a night or a weekend? Get back to romantic behaviour (see page 140). Take up a physical hobby together so that you are bodily active with each other doing something non-genital. Get out a video that will make you laugh. In other words do anything that enlivens your life together as a couple. Learn from your friends by observing how they have fun.

All this, together with your increasing intimacy should, with luck, start to create real joy – that deep sense of aliveness, wholeness and spontaneity which enables you to get in touch, however fleetingly, with your soul and possibly that of your partner. Relax and play together; make planned times for fun so that things actually happen; seek spontaneous fun in unlikely situations; get involved in something socially within the community or at one of the children's schools and so on. Many of us are so absorbed in the 'big things' of life that we lose sight of the small ones, yet it is usually in such things that joy is to be found.

Intimacy enables most couples to discover delight and joy in situations that would have previously appeared boring, dull or ordinary. And given that much of life is, by definition, ordinary this is no mean advantage to becoming more intimate. Delight and joy in life's ordinariness soon spreads to the bedroom and sex becomes more fun and relaxed.

COMMITMENT

This rather old-fashioned word is coming back into its own in the 1990s. It used to be something that many people sought to avoid but public attitudes have changed. Perhaps alternative life-styles without commitment have been found wanting; perhaps AIDS has made sexual caution more necessary; I do not know. But I do know that ten or fifteen years ago I had problems 'selling' commitment and today I do not. Perhaps today people can give themselves permission to enjoy commitment in relatively short-lived relationships whereas until recently the word was usually associated with a lifelong marriage.

Commitment does not just involve sex, however. It means making a promise to dedicate ourselves to our relationship and its future. Making such a commitment involves two processes. The first is a one-off decision to make this particular partnership special and is the sort of commitment we make when we decide to pair up in the first place. The other is an on-going commitment that we renew every day: the sort of commitment that takes nothing for granted, keeps us on our toes and ensures that we do not get lazy.

When we make a commitment to our partner we also make one to ourselves. In a sense this is the more important one because our partner cannot live our life for us. Only we can commit ourselves to growth and self-development. We can commit ourselves to one another too by agreeing to try to make the relationship work and to stick at it even when things are going badly.

All of this means putting effort, time and energy into our commitment, whether it is to ourselves or our partnership, and this means there will be a cost. Whenever I discuss commitment with couples they begin to count the cost. Early on in a relationship it can seem unacceptably high. As intimacy grows, though, and the commitment begins to pay off they say that what seemed a great price at first was in fact the best investment they had ever made.

When I address the acceptance of commitment clinically with couples we usually come across the issue of 'self' fairly early on. Being committed means giving up certain things that we would otherwise have done had we not been in such a relationship. Of course we also gain others that flow from the relationship itself. I always promise couples that, although it might not seem like it at the time, within a committed relationship one plus one can usually add up to at least three! We shall see on page 46 how concerns about freedom can get in the way of commitment but to some extent a voluntary surrender of some of our freedom is the very basis of any enduring, committed relationship. The fact that we are able to make such an apparent sacrifice, not for our partner, as is often claimed, but for the relationship, is the very bedrock of success in intimacy together.

In practical terms, commitment to a relationship involves sexual fidelity; making time for one another; behaving in specific ways that promote the relationship; agreeing, however implicitly, that this commitment is not just for a week or two but for a very long time, possibly for ever; and much more. Once basic agreements on these areas have been negotiated the relationship can weather many storms, disagreements and traumas from within and without because the deal that has been struck is presumed to be a lasting one. This is the 'till death us do part' part of the marriage ceremony and for many it still has great appeal.

All this might sound rather idealistic but in practice it is not. In daily life it comes down to balancing the many commitments we have to friends, parents, children, work, hobbies, and so on in such a way that our main commitment, to our relationship, remains paramount. Without this central commitment the other matters give us little joy or lasting satisfaction. I have known many wealthy people who apparently have everything the material world can give. Yet when they cannot sustain a committed relationship most of them feel impoverished at a soul level for which their material wealth can never compensate.

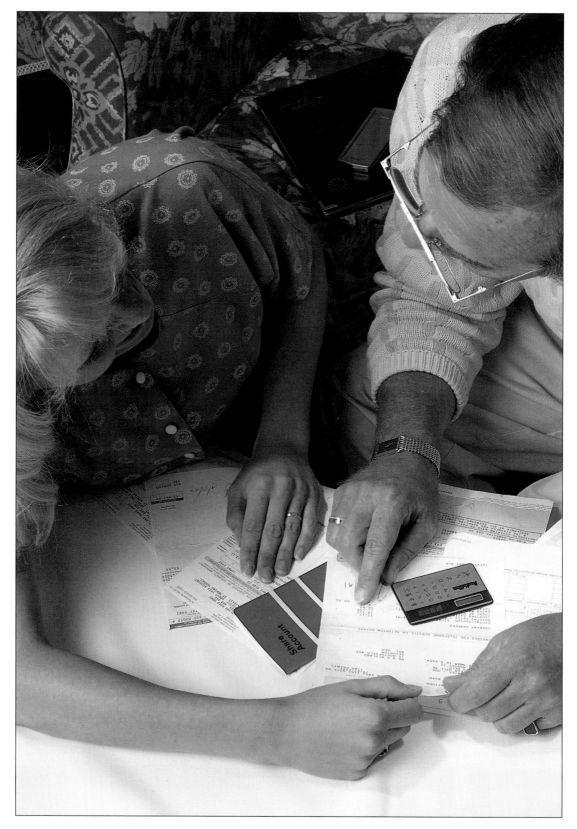

I find, both personally and professionally, that to keep one's commitment alive it helps to say something out loud about it. Actually declare something to your partner. Try to avoid making promises that you cannot or will not keep. Try to become aware of the patterns in your relationship that disable your ability to feel committed, and talk them through. Ask yourself what it would take to break up your relationship. If you can think of nothing then you do indeed have a durable commitment. You will also be very unusual!

However we see commitment and its value to us, it is certainly a good antidote to life's crises. We all have crises in our lives. Some are major and others trivial; some involve one of us personally and others involve the partnership as a unit. but whatever the crisis, our commitment must be to the future life of our relationship, not to its demise. A full and total commitment allows us to cope with even major crises. A small commitment waterproofs us very little against the travails of life and the pressures inherent in modern relationships.

The problem is that none of us can ever swear that we will give 100 per cent commitment all the time. After all, as we have seen, there are often many areas of life that demand their own particular commitments from us. This can be a real problem for those starting out in a new relationship, be it at twenty or sixty. How can we know with certainty that we will be able to remain totally committed in any situation?

The answer, of course, is that we cannot know. Yet in this 'not knowing' we still have to commit ourselves in faith. This in turn tells our lover that we are prepared to risk our love, our life, our time, our energy, our sexuality and so on *for the relationship*. We do not do it for our partner. Many people find this a troublesome concept. Women especially say things like 'I'd do anything for him'. For the person referred to in such a statement the pressures are high. Sometimes far too high. Whilst it might sound romantic to promise total commitment to our *partner* I find that it is more realistic and far more growthful to make the promise to the relationship. The partnership, after all, includes ourselves and we do not, therefore, feel hard done by as we 'sacrifice' various freedoms, or whatever, 'for our partner'. Out of a ready and conscious willingness we now make sacrifices for the relationship in the faith that all three of us – partner, self and relationship – will benefit. Commitment now becomes a royal road to freedom rather than the cage it at first appeared to be. Such commitment brings lasting joy.

The time to make a commitment, however, is not when we are head over heels in love, or when we are 'sick with love'. Being 'in love' is no reason to settle down and embark upon a long-term relationship. Arguably it is the very worst time to do so. Making a commitment intelligently means having sufficient knowledge of oneself and one's lover to be able realistically to start out on a journey that has at least

Commitment to a relationship goes way beyond sexual fidelity. It involves taking mutual responsibility for mundane, everyday things that have to be done no matter what is happening sexually. Many a couple's sexual life founders when they try to keep bedroom and outside world apart.

a fair chance of success. It is for this reason that I suggest to couples that they get the powerful drug called sex out of their veins before they even consider setting out on a committed relationship. Once we emerge from the unreal state of being 'in love' we can commit ourselves to something of greater depth and permanence as we see our beloved not as a reflection of our own narcissistic self but as he or she really is. With this kind of knowledge we can then decide whether or not we want to make a commitment that will lovingly bind us together.

PERSONAL FREEDOM

In recent decades much has been written and said about personal freedom. Yet in many cultures around the world the very concept seems crazy. Such peoples live and work for one another as a community and as an extension of their natural environment. In contrast, and there is no room in a book such as this to go into the many, complex reasons why, we in the West have come to prize personal freedom, or what we perceive it to be.

It is often said that males value their personal freedom more than do females and that one of the reasons that they are 'not much good at being intimate' is because it seems to encroach on this freedom to act in the way they want. Women, on the other hand, are said not to value personal freedom as much because they would rather emphasize their connection with others.

Neither stereotype is correct in any absolute sense. It is all a matter of degree. Many people I see talk about how free they will be once they are divorced but what they mean by the word 'free' varies a lot. To women it often means freedom to be independent and autonomous whereas to men it often signifies 'less of a tie', 'being less trapped' or 'having fewer responsibilities'. The freedom such women talk of is the reduction in responsibility for their husbands' emotions and largely comes from inside the woman. The freedom of which men talk is juxtaposed with pressures that are largely external: the restraining forces of confinement that being pair-bonded to another brings.

I have for some years been counselling young people who are about to get married. A recurring theme is that of freedom. Indeed, the vast exodus from marriage in recent years and the search for alternatives that appear to 'trap' the participants less is a feature of modern pair-bonding. Unfortunately, most people have never really thought much about freedom. When I discuss this issue with couples it is clear that the *idea* of freedom is much more attractive than the reality.

To cut a long story short, most thinking people soon come to realize that personal freedom has very little to do with being free from what others do to us; but it has everything to do with how free we are to take responsibility for ourselves and to become self-fulfilled. No matter what life-style we adopt with another human being, we always have to contend with the issues I have looked at in this part of the book. They are, after all, at the heart of all human interactions, whatever the label. Unhappily, many people misuse marriage and other long-term arrangements as they try to escape from pain in the world. Their expectations cannot then be met because they see marriage as 'the answer' to life's imperfections: a final solution rather than a simple beginning. Anyone who escapes into a one-to-one relationship is soon disillusioned. The 'closeness' that they think they need is soon shown up for the sham it is and they either cannot or choose not to be intimate. This sort of 'freedom' to escape from the single life into coupledom is as fruitless as the reverse: the flight to the 'freedom' of divorce. Alas, most people I deal with soon find that unless they were seeking freedom from pathological behaviour in their spouse (such as long-term criminality, addictions, physical abuse and so on) their life once 'free' often seems pointless and fruitless.

Although I am often accused of over-selling coupledom, I cannot but conclude from years of looking carefully at many life-styles that the best hope most of us have of achieving self-knowledge and intimacy with people in general is to work at creating and maintaining a one-to-one partnership, with or without marriage. Such self-direction and insight comes only with knowing more about oneself than about one's partner. The more we know about ourselves the better partner we make. So in this sense building a significant relationship with another frees us up to be more ourselves and then, paradoxically, to be more for others.

This sort of freedom allows us to be separate and yet not to have to leave. The battle that rages in most of us between our need to belong and our need to be separate can thus be calmed as both needs are met in the same setting. As we live together it is inevitable that the world will change and that we as individuals will change as well. Couples seeking freedom from the pains of such change by leaving and looking for another relationship simply take their itchy-footed search for freedom elsewhere, usually to repeat the stresses and dissatisfactions that go with it. Being able to find emotional space within a relationship and yet maintain that bond must be one of the greatest freedoms that human beings can experience.

Many people I see find it hard to cope with such normal and inevitable distancing. Yet times spent apart doing our own things usually enrich an intimate relationship as the 'absent' one brings seedcorn back into the partnership on his or her return. There is a lot of freedom in all this.

Whenever people complain to me that marriage is like a cage I try to get them to discover how they could alter their perception of this 'reality' by seeing the bars as widely spaced and the cage as very large. Given that we are all caged to some extent in the sense that society and our own unconscious trap us all, any concept of freedom is somewhat notional. As I work through these issues with couples they often accuse me of making matters worse by leading them to believe that they will have fewer freedoms. Unfortunately, the proof of the matter only comes with practice, and this calls for trust and faith in both myself and their partner.

Many of us seek and find freedom outside our loving relationship. This can be very healthy. No marriage or living-together arrangement can survive if we cling to each other in a dependent, desperate way. It is just too saccharine and disables growth. Paid work can be the main source of such freedom for some but so too can bringing up a family or being a housewife who is active in the community. It should not be forgotten that some surveys claim that about three-quarters of the population are dissatisfied with their jobs; and others find that women based at home with their families fare better than those who are employed full time in salaried work. Today's third-wave feminist appreciates the difference between men and women and relishes the wide range of options open to her. She is more able to choose to stay at home; breast-feed her babies; be a whole-hearted mother, and so on than many of her earlier feminist sisters. This is indeed a freedom, freedom from having to go along with the perceived wisdom of the previous generation's thinking. Freedom to be truly herself.

Lastly, let us not forget that many a relationship has been damaged by what I would call too much freedom. We all need boundaries within which to operate and this is especially true of intimate partnerships at any stage of life. Just as when we are tiny we need to know that our parents set boundaries within which we can be ourselves, the same applies to the raging teenager. Lessons learned at these stages of life translate into our one-to-one partnerships and few of us could happily exist, let alone thrive, in one which was based on total freedom. Agreeing the boundaries, however, can be a major task for any dedicated couple and a commitment to them is what helps successful partnerships survive and grow. In this sense George Orwell was right when he claimed that 'freedom is slavery'.

RETHINKING DEPENDENCY

Any journey towards greater intimacy soon involves tackling the issue of dependency. By and large we bring boys up to be 'independent' and girls to be somewhat 'dependent'. When working with couples for whom all this is a problem I usually start out by exploring the concept of healthy dependency in babies and children. This is vital to building the sort of courage and security that enables a child to experiment with independence. Only when this new state has been mastered and real lessons learned can an adult embark on a life of inter-dependence with another. All too often people try to put the cart before the horse.

On balance it is probably fair to say that most males regard independence as a commodity worth having, that this is how they want to be. To a man, independence means freedom, power, self-sufficiency and happiness. To females, however, it often means feeling unloved and alone and a lack of intimacy. Most women know intellectually that being independent has its uses but when I raise the issue of 'independent women' females think negatively of hard-bitten women who cannot relate to others intimately. This is a stereotype that, even today, people of both sexes find unattractive.

Generally, then, men think that independence is largely good and women that it is somewhat bad. Paradoxically, though, if you ask men whether or not they would marry again if anything happened to their wife the vast majority say that they would. As we see on page 76 marriage suits and advantages men more than it does women so this response is hardly surprising. If women are asked the same question, however, about half say that they would not marry again. Understandable,

For many men intimacy is inextricably linked with negative notions of dependency. They fear that to be truly intimate they have to return to unhealthy feelings of childhood dependency. Truly intimate couples, though, know how to separate the two and enjoy both in different ways.

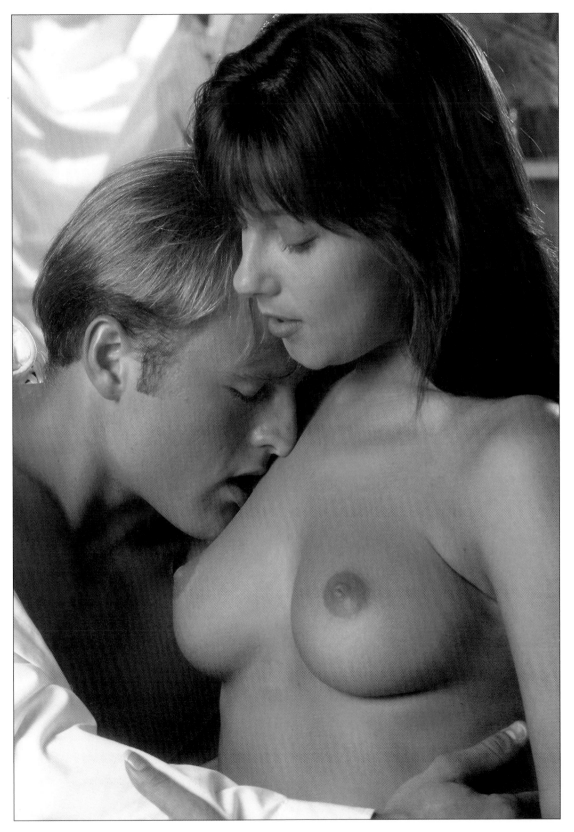

perhaps, given that women put much more into marriage and that for many it is a one-way street they regret having travelled. They have paid too heavy a price.

All this at first seems contradictory. How can men who prize independence so highly want marriage so much; whereas women who value dependency want to get out of it, or at least not to repeat it? The problem is that because men have largely been financially independent for so long we have come to believe that they are emotionally independent too. This is not the case. Many women know this and experience it in their everyday lives. I asked one woman how many children she had. She answered, 'Four', in a knee-jerk way. Then quickly added, 'That's including my husband, of course.' She was being honest, not stringing me along.

Men then come to see their partner as a sort of emotional service centre and look to their woman to answer their needs in this area of life. They also expect their partner to affirm them and facilitate emotional expression in a way that other areas of their life do not. Most men say that they cannot risk another man seeing them hurting or 'weak' but that this is acceptable with a woman because this is 'women's stuff'. So it is that women become the sole emotional support for their men. Indeed, they often provide *all* the emotional business within the relationship as a unit. This suits men but leaves women feeling short-changed. All this works well at one level, however, because the woman knows that her man is tied to her for this service and that she offers a priceless commodity. *She* pays a price too, though, especially in a relationship in which the traffic is one-way.

A man tied to a sole source of emotional intimacy not only feels good, however, he also feels bad because there is always the possibility that what he desires so much could be removed from him, as happened in childhood with the loss of his mother. This is why so many men deny their dependency on their partner with a ferocity that is clearly defensive at an unconscious level. The trouble with this for the couple wanting more intimacy is that it is an unequal equation. Intimacy cannot develop between two people who are unequal in any fundamental way.

We saw on page 20 how all this starts to come about in childhood but any couple that wants to build more intimacy successfully has to start on a different road. Women have to give up their role of emotional saviour and men must start to take responsibility for their own innermost selves. Women with whom I discuss this are often loath to let go of their 'emotional rescuer' role. This is because it has given them considerable power. Most men, too, do not greatly encourage their woman to let go of the emotional reins, knowing at some deep level that their inner security and ability to live in a hostile world depend upon having a woman at their side. Laziness is also to blame: many men prefer someone else to take responsibility for the difficult task of dealing with emotions.

Until a couple can clearly see the game they are playing in this area of life it is impossible for either of them to change and develop their intimate life as equals, taking responsibility for themselves first and then for one another. This calls for changes in thinking about emotional and financial dependency. More women are still financially dependent on their man than the other way around; and most men are hugely dependent on their women emotionally. For success, though, both have to yield some of the 'power' that these big weapons give them. In this journey there are bound to be hiccups as each learns to grow up and use this power for the benefit of the relationship rather than themselves. Both sexes need to recognize when it is appropriate to be dependent on the other and then to do deals with one another so that there is a balance of advantage to both. Sometimes a woman might feel 'weak' and 'dependent' in material and financial areas of life but at some other time her man will experience exactly the same disadvantages in the emotional zone. In his striving for financial 'power' and so-called independence a man is usually trying to armour himself against the world and its pains by 'doing' and 'winning' just in case he cannot rely on his partner to be there for him when he needs simply to 'be'. Much male autonomy and so-called independence is unconscious whistling in the dark. Many men with whom I discuss this say that deep down they feel as if they were a little boy some, or even much, of the time. Indeed for many this is a way of life that is all too apparent to them. Some of the most macho men I know are in fact hurting inside like vulnerable little boys, while trying to be self-contained and denying their reliance on 'bloody females'.

Many women, on the other hand, are so addicted to attachment and relationship that they will damage themselves rather than be without either or both. The little girl who turned to her father to experience her 'difference' from her mother now turns to her lover. Alas, his response often infantilizes her and this, added to the responses of the world at large, makes her despair (see page 24).

Whether this need for attachment, perfectly healthy in itself, is perceived in another way – as an unhealthy need for dependency – is very much in the eyes of the beholder. Attachment and dependency are not the same. We can remain attached to someone on whom we are no longer dependent. This often happens after divorce. Similarly, we can be dependent on someone to whom we are not attached. Perhaps if more couples understood the difference between attachment and dependency more might be able to find intimacy. Most women are crying out for attachment yet it would be cruel to suggest that because of this they are unhealthily dependent. Women's craving for attachment can sometimes appear to men to be claustrophobic and clinging and at its worst can actually drive men away from intimacy. Perhaps if we could all see that this is as misleading as the male myth of independence we would all get on better. Men, too, crave attachment, as can be seen by the way so many fall apart after divorce.

Perhaps one of the greatest fears that men have in encouraging their woman to be less unhealthily dependent is that once their woman is free within herself they might be abandoned. This harks back to childhood when fears of being left by mother were truly terrifying. So it is that many men unconsciously encourage their wife's unhealthy dependency. At the conscious level, such men realize that their woman's independence brings them and the relationship huge benefits but deep down in the unconscious they feel as if they were a little child about to be abandoned. Until this deep pain and fear can be addressed and lived through there is no hope for such a couple to experience true intimacy. If, however, both partners can come to accept their own weaknesses and fears of loss as part of the human condition that they both have to face in their own way, then unconscious games can be kept to a minimum and real growth towards intimacy can follow.

THE RESCUER–VICTIM–TYRANT TRIANGLE

Whole books have been written about this complex and fascinating subject yet I can make only brief reference to it here. It is, however, a matter well worth exploring by all couples who are trying to make their relationship more intimate. And it is a potential minefield of which we should all be aware.

Within all of us there are fragments of many different types of personality. None of us is all one thing or another. Although there are hundreds of character traits that manifest themselves in human beings, three main ones seem persistently to get in the way of intimacy. These unconscious traits are rescuing, being a victim and being tyrannical or punitive. Most people exhibit at least one of these traits; for some, one is very obviously a dominant behaviour style. We all seek to be a *rescuer* to somebody in however subtle and unwitting a way; we all behave and feel like *victims* in certain circumstances; and most of us can act *tyrannically* or punitively towards those we love.

I will start with rescuers as they are thick on the ground. Many more are female than male, and they tend to have the following characteristics. They focus on the ills of others rather than their own; they quickly home in on anyone who needs fixing, advising or helping and take them over; they cannot keep away from other people's struggles with their pain: they move in and try to help; they find difficulty in sharing their own woundedness, especially with others they perceive to be wounded; and lastly, they become known as people who are always 'together' and reliable. In short, they can appear somewhat 'saintly'.

Such an 'overfunctioning' individual usually pairs with someone who is an 'underfunctioner' or victim. To all the world the rescuer appears to be the stronger one who supports his or her partner and everybody else who has a problem. In fact he or she is just as wounded as other people, often much more so. Rescuers spend much of their time and effort turning their psychic spotlight outwards in order to avoid the pain of what they would discover if they were to turn it inwards. Rescuing others is a socially acceptable way of avoiding contact with their innermost selves.

Victims feel negative about themselves a lot of the time. They think others feel badly about them; turn their pains inwards and become angry and depressed; feel they are unworthy of improvements in their lives; unconsciously seek out rescuers to help them cope with life; and generally hide their form of woundedness in inertia. They have a magnetic attraction for rescuers.

The tyrant within us seeks to punish others or ourselves. We project our own annoyance and fury at ourselves on to those around us to make them suffer. We suffer too by doing so.

Rescuing, being a victim or a tyrant are all forms of unconscious defence which, to some extent, we all need. When things get out of balance, however, and we

---

We all want to be loving and compassionate when our partner is 'down',
but it is essential to be aware of any hidden 'rescuer' or 'victim' business
that might be going on underneath the surface.

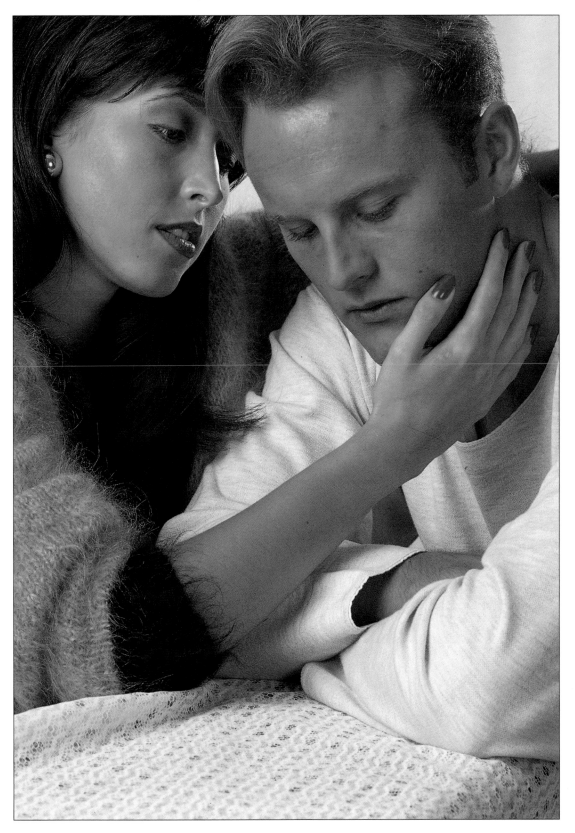

misuse one or other mode by making it our main way of dealing with reality, then we suffer and cannot create intimate relationships. Most people function predominantly in one or more of these ways and some whom I see are lost in the world of one or another system. Thinking of these three defences as a triangle helps us to see how it is that we tend to move from one to another. When I see a compulsive rescuer, therefore, we first address the original wounds and pains against which this rescuing is a defence. If this is not done the individual slips easily into victim or punitive mode. Similarly, if we deprive a victim of his or her opportunity to continue in this style of behaviour he or she can turn into a tyrant or a rescuer: anything to avoid the pain of facing the original hurts that created the defences in the first place.

Although it is easy to see that those who behave in a punitive way to their partner are not candidates for intimacy, the other two models are much more difficult to deal with because rescuers are so 'nice' and victims such 'poor little things'. If I am to be a rescuer, however, you have to become a victim or I will not have a role to play; and you may not want to be a victim any more. I see this repeatedly in my work with couples. A woman may have started off in married life quite happy to be 'punished' in various unconscious and subtle ways, but in her thirties she may want to change this relationship model. As she starts to become her own person and refuses to play victim to his rescuer the sparks fly and he can become punitive or even a 'poor little victim' himself. Either partner can start off in one corner of the triangle while pressure for change from one of the other corners, occupied by their mate, shifts the whole balance of the system. This can create havoc for the unaware couple.

It is not difficult to see that someone who is being cast by their partner's unconscious to fit any of these roles will be highly unlikely to feel safe enough to be truly intimate. Such couples are often very 'close'. In fact the nature of their unconscious game means that they are usually over-close, but this does not make for intimacy. Indeed it is the enemy of intimacy.

Any couple working on themselves and trying to become more 'conscious' should attempt to become aware of how they stand in this triangle of defences. Listen to what others say about you, both individually and as a couple; hear what your partner says when he or she is upset about your behaviour or attitudes; talk through together how you think you unconsciously created this unhelpful system and try to modify your behaviour and attitudes with one another's help. I say this advisedly because many of the couples I hear complaining about a lack of intimacy are deeply enmeshed in this triangle yet make all kinds of excuses to continue with it. This is because, although it clearly does them few favours, it at least feels familiar. Unless we can tackle the original matters that caused the defences to be built in the first place, and this can be tricky or impossible without professional help, the best we can do is to try to modify our behaviour towards our partner and ourselves in a way that stops the harmful triangle growing. Other efforts at increasing intimacy can then make inroads into our defences; and as we come to feel safer we need these defences less. In this way even quite hardened rescuers, victims or tyrants can find healing within their one-to-one relationship.

RAGE AND ANGER

There can be few emotions more damaging to intimacy between partners than hidden rage and anger. To me, as a working therapist, the two are closely related but not quite the same. Anger is often perfectly reasonable and even desirable, given that the world contains people and events that make us angry. Much of the anger we feel arises as a result of issues of which we are consciously aware in the present. Much anger can be dealt with at this level either by ourselves, our partner or both of us.

If, however, the real cause of the anger comes from deep inside us, from our unconscious, then we may project our old responses to a previous source of anger on to the screen that is our partner. This unconscious origin is almost always the source of true *rage*. Once we get out of control and really rage at someone, it is no longer ourselves in the here-and-now behaving in this way but an old voice that was not heard at some distant time in the past. My work with regression suggests that all true rage originates from ancient times in our personal history, often from the cradle and sometimes even from within the womb itself.

Not all anger, however, is destructive or negative in its outcome. Many good works and positive outcomes originate from an individual or group who are so angry over a particular issue that they are moved to act, often out of compassion. The key part of this word is 'passion'. When we are being compassionate in this context we are using anger constructively. When our anger is unfocused and usually when we rage we return to being a hurting baby or child and can do little or no constructive work for ourselves, our relationship or indeed anyone else.

In our culture many of us have become used to turning our anger inwards for fear of hurting others or becoming unacceptable to them or ourselves. This almost never produces anything but pain, either at the time or later. A common sort of personality is the passive-aggressive individual who seems angelic on the outside and is generally thought of as a 'really nice person'. I am wary of such people right from the start and know from experience that it is only a matter of hours in therapy before the real individual comes out from behind the mask to reveal himself or herself for the angry or even raging soul that he or she is. I use the word 'soul' advisedly because I find that most of these individuals are suffering neither from a mental illness, nor from the depression that so many manifest outwardly, but from a deep soul sickness that strikes at the very core of their being.

The problem with *showing* anger is that it usually makes others feel we are being hostile and aggressive to *them*, even if we are not; and that it makes us feel awkward, or worse, as we perceive that at least some of our anger is directed at ourselves. We also unconsciously know exactly whom the anger or rage is really aimed at from our past and this in itself makes us feel uncomfortable or even desperate. Small wonder then that most of us avoid anger much of the time and certainly try to keep well away from rage. All this avoidance works tolerably well in normal social interactions but for the couple seeking intimacy it is a disaster.

No really intimate relationship can be based on hidden anger and rage. One of the main reasons for this is that the sorts of armour required to keep the anger

Continued on page 58

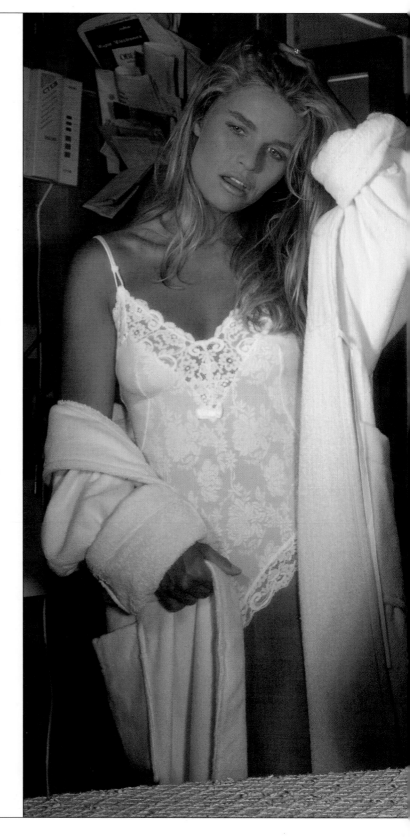

Rage is a very human emotion that some men show in sexual settings. Almost all such fury dates from way back in childhood but emerges to haunt both him and his partner in the here-and-now. If we can successfully separate out old, often primitive, anger from what is really happening now we can avoid burdening our lover with our psychological baggage.

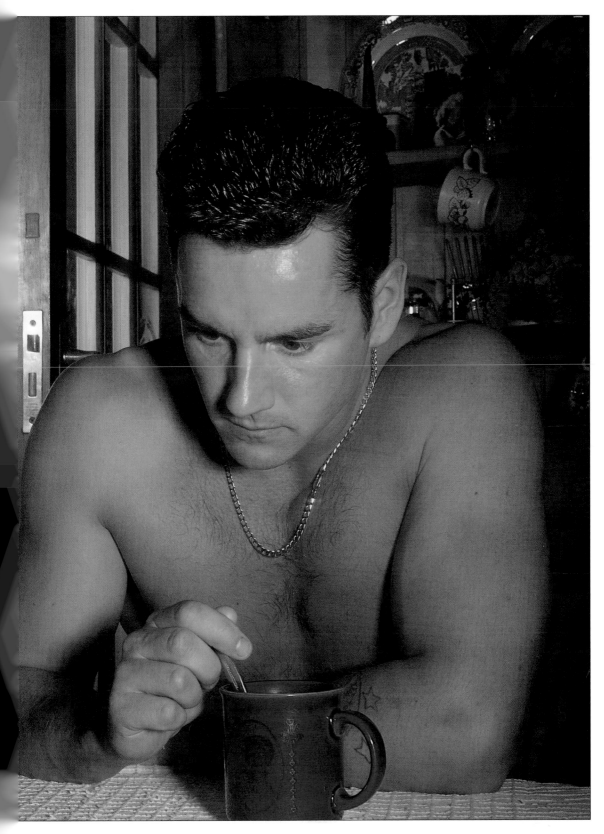

inside us also serve us badly in our quest for intimacy. Our bodily and psychic armour is not clever enough to filter things out selectively. The defences that help us keep our rage and anger under control also disable us by holding back our more constructive passionate emotions and intimacy once more suffers as a result. Real people being truly themselves are open to their passions (I do not mean only their sexual ones). Many people talk about the released creativity at home, work and in the family once they have dealt with their anger and rage. They soon see how their armour plating has kept back *all* passion, not just their anger.

So what can be done about this? First of all, though it might seem simplistic, I ask couples to acknowledge that there are things in life generally and in their relationship in particular that really infuriate them. When you begin exploring this as a couple start off with easy areas that do not involve either of you as a pair. Use your empathic listening skills (see page 129) really to hear what your partner is saying. Afterwards reflect back on what you think you have heard.

At this stage you will probably feel confident enough to move on to things about your partner that upset you. Try not to attack or generalize, avoiding phrases such as, 'You always do . . .'; 'Why is it that you never . . . ?' Keep away from all sweeping statements about gender, such as 'Women are all the same . . .'. Really listen, just as you did on the other subjects and try to see what is at the heart of your partner's anger. It could well be that your partner does not know. This gives you you an opportunity to sit down and work through some possible origins for the anger, using what you know about one another and your respective pasts and present difficulties (see page 133).

The secret of making all this work is what therapists call 'containment'. In this the listening partner (the one not expressing the anger) puts his or her ego to one side and stops being concerned with how justified the cause of the anger is; does not seek to deny the partner's feeling; and does not jump in with explanations but simply hears what is said acting almost like a container into which the partner is pouring his or her anger. When we behave in this way we do not have to own our partner's anger or rage: after all it belongs to our partner, not to us. We do not even have to agree. The 'container' does not have to interact with the material being poured into it; all it has to do is to hold it against the day when the owner can come back and retrieve it. It is a sort of emotional left-luggage facility. Our only task as listener is to acknowledge that our partner is angry and that this anger or rage is real to him or her and entirely justified at that time. I say 'at that time' because a common scenario is for one partner to rage at the other, then quickly calm down and apologize for doing so in such an unjustifiable way. Such an individual realizes at some level that the outburst had little or nothing to do with his or her partner directly. It also becomes clear that the partner was being used as a surface on to which to project underlying rage. Perhaps, as is often the case, the partner consciously or unwittingly pressed a button to set the projector going.

This sort of mirroring and containing calls for some rules if it is to be successful. First, no one must hit their partner or do any physical damage to them. Second, it must be agreed that no one leaves the room until the issue has been adequately heard through. I have known people, especially females, who, having been wound up by a partner who was unable or unwilling to be empathic, storm out of the room or home and try to kill themselves. Lastly, it makes sense to limit your comments to descriptions of events rather than assassinating your partner's personality. For example, it is far better to say, 'I hate the way you go and spend money on new clothes when you know we're in trouble with the bank', than, 'You are a money-grabbing bitch spending all the money when I slave so hard to earn it'.

This sort of containment creates a healthy environment in which we can express anger safely. The underlying issues can then often be dealt with by quiet and loving discussion once the heat has gone out of the situation. After all, we do not agree to *take on* our partner's anger, but simply to *contain* it. This means that once our partner is stable again emotionally and feels listened to, we can allow him or her to retrieve the emotions from the container and deal with them little by little in a helpful way. Most of us scare ourselves when we are very angry; simply having someone there who can hold on to some boundaries for us helps us feel safe enough to let the anger and rage out.

All of this works very well provided that we can keep our business and that of our partner separate. Troubles arise when our inner, hurting child starts to interact with that of our partner. The scene is now set for a re-enactment of pains for which neither of us has the answer. In such a state we can do one another terrible emotional harm. Any safety there may have been with boundary control is now lost and the potential for mutual and self-destruction is great. Given that we all choose one another (see page 35) with this potential in our unconscious it is hardly surprising that some of the worst anger and rage is to be found within relationships that have the greatest potential for intimacy.

This is a paradox that we all have to live with if we are to risk forming an intimate relationship with our beloved. The very material that attracts us and makes it possible for us to live together most of the time also has the capacity to explode in our faces unless we are acutely aware and have spent a long time working on the original sources of our anger and rage.

This is best done in a therapeutic relationship with someone to whom we are not attached romantically. It *can*, however, be done carefully over many years by the couple who can listen empathically and contain one another's anger while the owner deals with it. This latter point is vital. Time and again I hear women particularly say that they would like to be able to help their partner deal with his anger. Many of us of either gender are over-eager to rescue our partner from the pain of his or her anger and rage. When a couple is with me, and one of them is getting really angry in the safe haven of my consulting room, the other will sometimes start to caress the partner; start to cry; try to calm the partner down; or in other ways seek unconsciously to shut him or her up. This person is unwittingly hijacking his or her partner's anger. Clearly the angry one is never allowed to express rage, but until this sort of game takes place in front of a neutral observer, the couple never realizes that this is what they do. We cannot take our partner's pains away when he or she is angry, even, or perhaps especially, if the anger is aimed at us. Anger craves to be heard and expressed somehow.

There are few situations in life in which it is possible to feel sufficiently safe that we can do such vital work on ourselves. Our intimate, one-to-one relationship is probably the best opportunity that most of us have. Couples who express anger healthily, especially about one another, tell me that rather than falling out, as they had predicted, they grow hugely in their intimate life together. Many couples say that they make love best of all after being angry and feeling really listened to. The raging little baby or child within us desperately cries out for parenting and an intimate partner can provide this, not in a cloying way that stifles the anger or denies it, but in a way that says, 'I can see you're angry. I love you, not in spite of your anger, but because of it. In your anger you are being truly human and I *want* you to be truly human or how else can we hope to live and grow together?'

RESOLVING CONFLICT

In any one-to-one relationship, whether it is between parent and child, employer and employee or lover and beloved, there is one thing of which we can be sure: there will be conflict from time to time. No meaningful relationship between two human beings can avoid it, if only because we are all so different. One of the major barriers to intimacy between lovers is that they do not know how to prevent conflict in the first place and then cannot resolve it when it occurs.

Prevention is usually better than cure, so let us start here. Encouraging our partner is a good beginning. People in relationships in which frequent encouragement is the norm find that conflict is less common and that when it does occur the existing goodwill soon helps overcome the original source of the conflict. Setting aside time to share your feelings about the relationship also helps, as does being open about practical issues such as where each of you will be at any time, who will do what and so on. A lot of conflict occurs over a simple lack of communication such as who had agreed to get the supper ready that night.

Try to be as honest as you can about what your expectations are of any situation. Conflict often arises from unrealistic expectations in one or both parties. Try to resolve small issues as they occur. Nip problems in the bud so that they do not even get a chance to grow into real conflict. Many of the couples I see say that this takes a lot of courage at first as it appears to multiply conflict situations, but they soon come to see that saving things up until they cannot cope with them any more creates even bigger rows. Successful couples seem to be able to see conflict coming early and disarm it before it causes damage.

Try to take responsibility for your own psychological and emotional business in life rather than projecting it on to your lover. Most of us create conflict, albeit unconsciously, by dumping our own anxiety, fear, anger, frustration, sexual arousal, or whatever, on to our partner. Understandably, our partner does not want to own it and conflict occurs.

Conflict is inevitable in any relationship that matters. Unconsciously choosing someone with whom we have so much to fight about makes for sparks but it also creates opportunities to learn and change. Imagine never having a disagreement. Most of us would die of boredom as well as lose out on extending ourselves and our relationship.

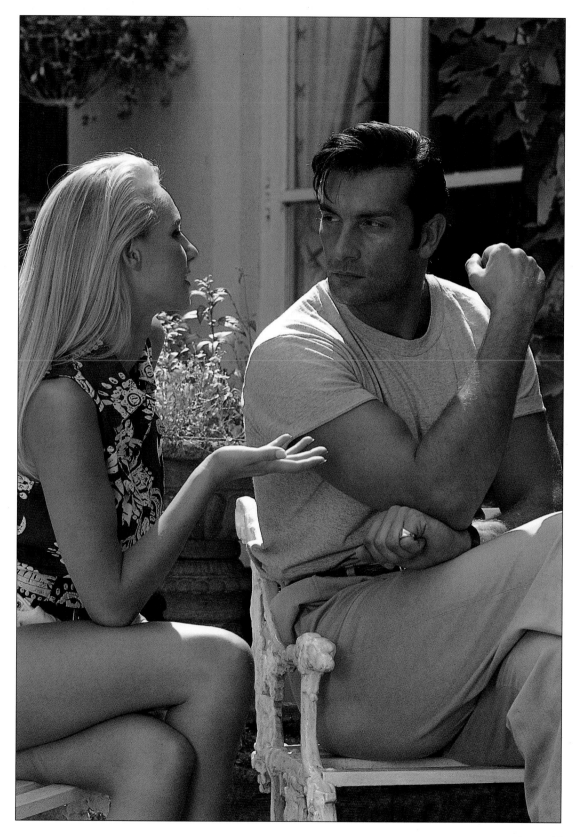

These simple preventives might work for you but it will not be easy – it never is, especially early on in a relationship when you are feeling your way with one another human being. In addition, you will need some skills and techniques for actually dealing with disagreement and conflict. The rule I generally work to is that all conflict should be sorted out to everyone's satisfaction, however incomplete, before the matter is left. I see couples who have seething conflicts that have been running for years. Needless to say, they cannot hope to be intimate against this sort of backdrop.

Early on in a relationship conflict is commonplace. This is probably inevitable. People who have been married for many years usually say that their most stressful time together was 'in the first few years as we were trying to find out about one another'. The problem for many young couples is working out how to cope with such disagreements; what is really worth creating a fuss over and what is not; and how to deal with real dilemmas when agreement appears to be impossible.

The trouble that almost all of us have when trying to handle conflict is mixing up fact with opinion. Most of us think that what we believe about any situation is 'fact'. We look at this in more detail on page 80. This then makes us 'right' and others 'wrong'. But as I know from my daily work, some couples cannot even agree on a simple matter such as how many times they had sex in the previous week, so even over 'facts' we can disagree terribly. Next come the problems inherent in the interpretation, conscious or unconscious, of these 'facts'. A man might well say to me rather gloomily, 'We made love *only* five times last month', whilst his partner says triumphantly, 'We made love *five* times last month!'. The same 'fact' can mean very different things to each partner.

Once we begin to tread the stony road of opinions we are in real trouble. To continue with the last couple, the man might now claim that, in his opinion, only two of the occasions were what he would call love-making at all. She had been uninterested, had not turned him on at all, and perhaps, on reflection, only one of the occasions could fairly have been called 'real sex'. His wife, on the other hand, thinking that she had been exactly what he wanted and, given her previous track record of sex every few weeks, felt she was being a real raver.

It is clear that our perceptions of what goes on in our relationship will sometimes vary greatly from those of our lover. But who is right? The answer is that we are both right . . . from our own viewpoint. No amount of arguing will prove one or the other to be right – or wrong. Listening empathically (see page 129), however, makes the other feel respected and, as we repeatedly see through the book, can throw valuable light on our unconscious if only we can be open enough. Being alive to what our lover's opinions are can therefore teach us a lot about ourselves.

This said, and even if we work well at trying to accommodate one another's viewpoints, there will always be areas of life that remain very difficult indeed. Moral issues such as sex outside marriage, abortion, certain 'perverse' sexual practices and so on come into this category. Such issues appear to be unresolvable because we have diametrically opposed views on which neither is prepared to compromise. The best thing here is to continue talking, and not, as many couples do, to go off in a huff, determined that they are on the side of the angels and that their partner is beyond redemption. Early on in a relationship you may just have to live with the fact that you do not agree on even quite major matters. This does not, as many young couples try to convince me, mean that the relationship is dead on the grounds of incompatibility; rather that it is very much alive *because* of the differences between you.

This brings us to the thorny subject of difference in general. We do not form an intimate relationship with someone who is a clone of ourselves. We would probably go mad if we did. By teaming up with someone different we certainly lay the foundation stones for rows and conflict but we also set ourselves up for growth.

Most of us like to think that we are very similar to our beloved and seek to play down difference and conflict. We do this for many reasons. Firstly, difference makes us feel separate and alone. Secondly, Western concepts of closeness make us minimize difference. Thirdly, being aware of difference makes us face up to the fact that one human being cannot hope to answer all our needs, and this is painful for many. Fourthly, day-to-day experience shows us that too much difference and conflict really does make life unpleasant and it is difficult to know where we should draw the line. Fifthly, looking at our differences makes us face our lover's weaknesses and indeed our own rather than living in a fantasy, romantic world where everything is rosy. Finally, difference and conflict can make us feel somehow 'wrong' (especially if our partner is 'right') in some sort of absolute sense, and this is uncomfortable.

The concept of compromise is often used to denigrate individuals or situations, yet all life is a compromise. None of us can have exactly what we want or need all the time and I have yet to meet a perfectly matched couple. Some young couples speak of having been misled in some way. What they thought they had 'bought' turns out to be a rather different product after some months or years. This can lead to self-blame as one partner, usually the woman in my clinical experience, berates herself for having made such an unsuitable choice.

Many couples fall at this stage of the race and condemn the partnership to death because they mistake difference for a fatal illness. Difference and the conflict it produces is, in fact, much more like the repeated challenge an allergy-inducing substance presents to the immune system: it results in greater immunity and helps resist future attacks. If, however, we see difference as fatal we fool ourselves and condemn ourselves to a life of seeking the perfect individual who will never cause us any grief. When I see couples who claim that they have found such a partner I ask myself why they are sitting in my consulting room. 'We never row', they claim. 'Why on earth not?', I reply, somewhat provocatively. Yet there they sit, unable to be intimate, having a boring and lack-lustre sex life and wondering how this can all be happening to 'such a nice couple' that never disagrees.

When dealing with difference and conflict in a relationship it is vital to bear in mind that whatever our tablets of stone appear to be telling us as they hang heavily around our neck, opinions, attitudes and experiences do change. Matters that today seem to be irreconcilable looked at six months or six years from now are often a source of mirth, disbelief or ridicule. The secret is not to behave as if today's conflict were likely to dog us for ever. 'You'll *never* understand'; 'I'll *never*

Continued on page 66

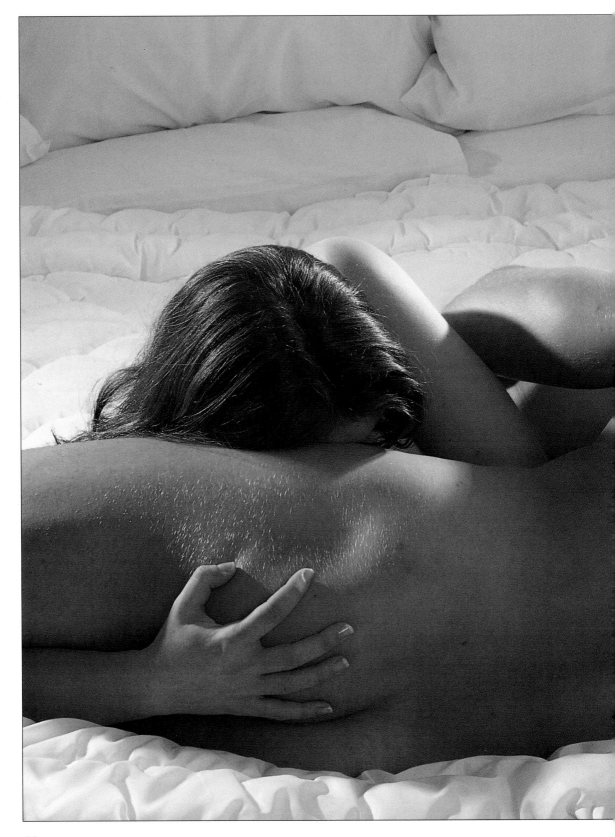

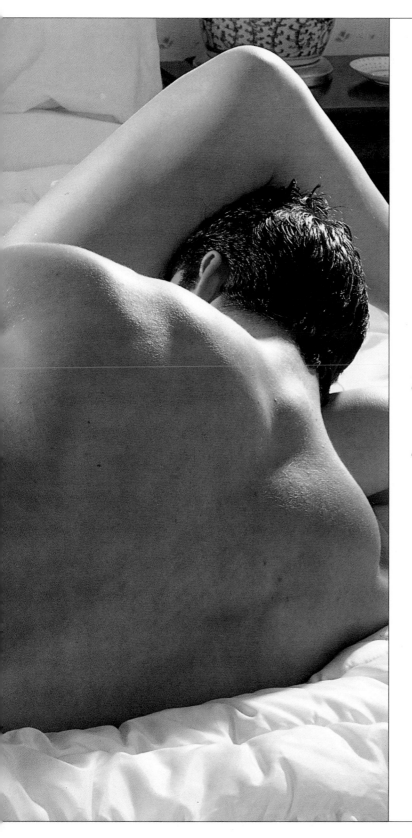

Trust and fidelity are an essential part of the intimate life. Of all love-making positions, this is the one that calls for the utmost trust. Not only does it say 'I trust you not to bite me!' but 'I trust you with the most delicate and private parts of my body.' In an age of safe sex it also means 'I trust that you will take responsibility for our joint sexual health.'

THE ART OF SEXUAL INTIMACY

change my mind about something as important as this'; 'You're so *stubborn*. Why can't you see it my way?', are just a few of the things we say when we feel right and righteous. The loss of dignity that occurs as a result of such exchanges and the corners into which we box ourselves weigh heavily on even a good relationship and make intimacy very difficult indeed. How much better to agree that we are bound to think differently about various matters; that our partner is just as likely to be right about things as we are; and that what really matters is that the relationship continues *because* of its differences rather than in spite of them.

TRUST AND FIDELITY

Trust is a commodity that is in short supply these days. In society in general and on a personal, couples level more and more people find it difficult to trust others. In the USA it is not uncommon to find pre-nuptial agreements; private detectives following partners who are thought to be errant; scant faith that a marriage will endure; and so on.

Trust can be difficult to define. Perhaps we can learn more about it by looking at its bedfellows: loyalty, fidelity, integrity and reliability. The trouble I find is that many people do not trust themselves; have poor experiences of untrustworthy adults from their childhood; are distrustful of many or even all of those they meet; and much more.

When trying to build an intimate life together the most basic foundation stone is trust. We have to believe that our partner can be trusted to be good to us and deal with us well when we are being open and truly ourselves. To some extent this calls for a degree of *predictability*, or we would be constantly wondering what was going to happen next; *dependability*, so that we can count on our partner should the need arise; and a *faith* that he or she will always be there and responsive to our needs. Human nature being the way it is, none of these commodities can be totally relied upon. I often find that individuals are wary of trusting their partners until they feel absolutely sure that they will not be let down. I sometimes have an uphill struggle persuading such people that eventually we simply have to take a deep breath and trust in faith or nothing will ever happen. We can never be *absolutely* sure that our partner will never let us down.

There are large numbers of everyday situations in which we need to be able to trust our partner, from money and children to emotional support and sex. At first these issues have to be negotiated individually but, as intimacy grows, the overall level of trust within the relationship covers all the activities in which a couple engages in their day-to-day life together.

When we trust a partner with whom we are sexually involved in an enduring relationship, it is often sexual fidelity that is most important. Being committed sexually and emotionally means that we do not devote our time, effort, energy, or sexuality to other situations or people; rather we dedicate their application in the sexual domain to our special and exclusive partner. Most couples come to some sort of agreement over time as to what their own particular thresholds are at which they define the start of infidelity. One couple's idea of acceptable flirtation is another's road to the divorce courts. Once such ground rules have been set, however, the intimate couple rarely, if ever, steps outside them unless one or other partner wants the relationship to end. Having said this, we are all human and can genuinely make mistakes or find ourselves vulnerable at a particular time or in a specific situation. It is then that the one-off transgression will need to be forgiven. Few couples break up valued, intimate relationships because of an isolated event. They have too much to lose and realize that one day they too might be tempted to stray. For those who have problems with trust dating from infancy and childhood, even the slightest sexual infidelity can spell the end of a relationship, but the vast majority of people today do not over-react in this way. Repeated unfaithfulness, however, calls for very different handling and can shatter the bond of trust so fundamentally that intimacy breaks down, often irretrievably.

This is no place to look at affairs in any detail but suffice it to say that an intimate couple always uses such an event to learn about themselves as individuals and as a pair. Recovery from such a loss of trust can take months or years. Some susceptible people find that although they can forgive their partner they can never forget and are presensitized to future transgressions. Sometimes such a lack of faith and harbouring of grudges so damages the re-establishing of intimacy that the errant partner wanders again as if unconsciously to fulfill his or her lover's prophesy that this will happen.

There are some steps that a couple can take to mend a loss of trust that has taken place. Firstly, it must be agreed that what has happened occurred because there was a breakdown in their relational system. I almost never see breaches of trust that are totally 'one person's fault'. Secondly, the one who has broken the trust must make strenuous efforts to be more dependable, loyal and committed or the partner will not believe that he or she is sorry or sees the breakdown as a problem to be remedied. The one who has been wronged must be willing to forgive, even if, early on, this feels impossible. Anger has to be vented and various pains from the present and the past must be acknowledged before forgiveness can even be considered. Simply to say, 'I forgive you' heals nothing and usually just papers over the cracks as it buries the painful emotions.

Lastly, we have to take responsibility for any of our actions that brought about the loss of trust, just as we do in other areas of life. At some level, however unconscious, we decided to violate the trust in our partnership. What made this likely and how we might have coped in other ways are both issues that have to be addressed, either alone within the partnership or with the help of a professional.

MEN AND INTIMACY

It is impossible to go very far in the discussion of intimacy without coming across the assertion that men are somehow disabled in this area of life. Therapists such as myself see countless women who claim that their men are almost totally crippled when it comes to intimacy. But is this so? Is it a fact that men have fewer intimate relationships than women do? Are men really disabled or unskilled in intimate matters? Do they, perhaps, need less intimacy than women? And, when all is said and done, does it matter to men, or their partners, if they are not much good at being intimate?

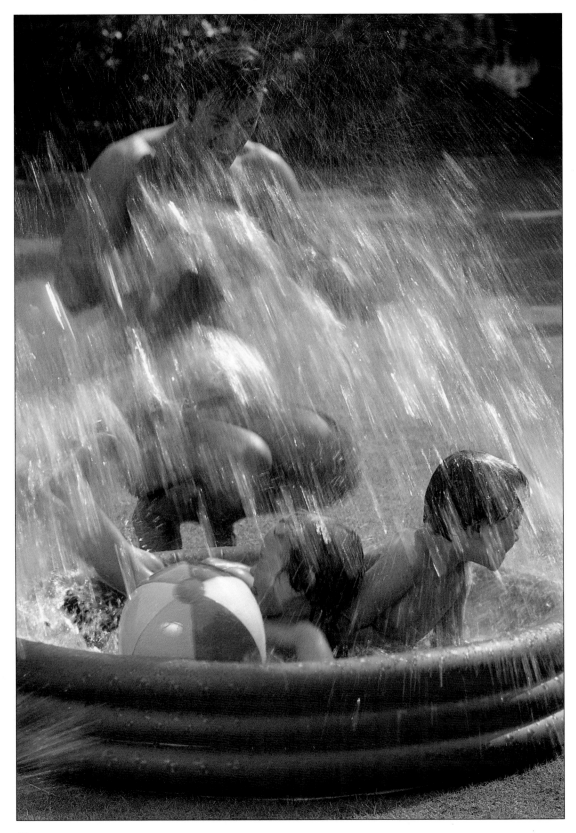

Let us start by looking at whether men actually have fewer intimate relationships than women do. No sooner do we embark on this subject than we come across the first of the paradoxes that plague this field of psychological research. The vast majority of studies, let alone individuals who express a view on the matter, claim that men take part in fewer intimate relationships than women do. Men, however, say that they like to belong to groups, often of like-minded males, and that to them this is a sort of intimacy. They can be truly themselves in the presence of others who are being truly *themselves*. The majority of women I discuss this with do not see this sort of affiliation as being at all intimate; at best, they say, it is close and often not even that. In this way the battle-lines are drawn in millions of homes the world over.

This mateship among men starts early in life. Almost all such relationships are based on shared activities and interests such as work, sport or hobbies. Males get together at all ages to *do* things together whereas females form intimate bonds to *be* things together. When I ask a man who his best friend is and with whom he is best able to be most intimate he will usually say that they are one and the same person, his partner. When women are asked the same question they usually say that it is their best girlfriend. There is also evidence that male friendships do not last as long as those of females. The average man has only a few friends (often less than three) with whom he is *ever* able to be vulnerable and intimate yet most women have a network of friends and acquaintances, and with several they feel safe enough to be really intimate.

If, in therapy, I ask a man who his best male friend is and when he last saw him the answer is often that they have not met up, let alone been intimate with one another, for many months or even longer. The same question put to his wife brings forth an answer that could not be more different: she is in almost constant contact with her intimate friend or friends.

There is considerable evidence that men's same-sex relationships tend to be much less intimate than women's do. For a start, most men reveal much less about themselves and their feelings than women do in all intimate relationships. There are many theories as to why this might be but I find that there is a considerable fear among men of being thought homosexual. One way that many men think they could be so labelled is if they were 'too close' or 'too intimate' emotionally with another man. There appears to be no such restriction among women; in fact, such a proposition would be considered laughable by the average woman. Also, in a largely self-centred culture such as in most Western societies, males are brought up from a very early age to see other males as potential or actual adversaries. They are taught that to be too open in their presence is to court disaster either at the time or in the future. These, and no doubt other culturally inbuilt circuits

---

Many men's first real adult experience of intimacy is when they become a father. Here they can learn to be truly themselves in the presence of others — their children — who are being truly themselves. *Separating all this from sexual intimacy can be a novel experience for many such men.*

unconsciously affect the very beginnings of any intimate relationship between males.

Having said this, some males do, in fact, have very intimate same-sex relationships, but they have to feel exceptionally safe in order to let their defences down. Alternatively they have to be very frightened, perhaps in the face of shared adversity. If the external concerns are greater or more pressing than the internal needs to maintain bullet-proof defences, then males *can* become intimate with one another just as women do.

Let us look now at some of the components of intimacy in daily life and see if men and women are in fact all that different. We saw at the start of the book that it is very difficult to define intimacy with any certainty and I suggested a working definition that seems to make sense to many of those I deal with. But however any individual would define intimacy there are several types of emotional business that almost everyone would include. Being able to talk about oneself and one's feelings comes high on the list when I discuss this with women. An ability to be empathic comes next; followed by an awareness of one's own feelings so that they *can* be expressed; and lastly the ability to express them verbally or non-verbally. All these are different and separate learned social skills. The possession of one does not necessarily mean an ability with another. People of either gender who have them all are perceived to be very able in intimate relationships.

As we have seen, there is far more to an intimate interaction between two people than simply what they *say*. Most couples, however, claim that they need to share at least some of their intimate feelings verbally at some stage. Many's the man I see who claims that he *is* very intimate, or feels he is, yet he simply does not talk about it. His wife sits there fuming, unable to understand how it is possible to be intimate at the level she wants and needs without actually talking. Most studies that have looked at this issue of self-disclosure have found that men do not reveal as much about themselves as women do in any setting, intimate or not; and when men do speak at this level they hide their weaknesses, whereas women hide their strengths.

This issue of control is important in intimate relationships between the sexes. The battle for power and control is ever-present at one level or another for much of the time in almost all man-woman relationships that are not deeply intimate. The truly intimate couple does not indulge in this energy-sapping game, but then such couples are probably few and far between. There can be little doubt that feelings, whether they are expressed openly or not, are a major part of being human. As far as we can possibly know, it is our feelings that distinguish us from other animate and inanimate objects. This means that whoever 'controls' this zone of life has considerable power and influence.

It is generally accepted in Western society that women have more power and control in this area. Indeed it could be said that until fairly recently they had so little control in most fields of life that they clung on to their influence in the emotional sphere rather doggedly. Many men over the years have told me that they dared not become too involved in emotional matters within the family because this was their wife's territory. And indeed it is my experience that many women, though perhaps this is less so in the last few years, hold the emotional baby very close to their bosom and are in fact quite resistant to letting it go.

So it is that most men see feelings as being 'women's business', as indeed do most women. In many marriages the man unwittingly hands over the management of emotional transactions within the relationship and family to his partner because she is better at it; or because, some argue, there has to be a division of labour in any working partnership and he would rather do the finances, mow the lawn and look after the car. Whether this is a fair distribution, though, is open to debate. Most women find dealing with emotional issues much more draining than do their partners with their car maintenance.

In many relationships, the woman wants her man to be more capable when it comes to self-disclosure: and indeed all the other facets of the intimate life. She is, however, usually unaware as to how she disables him by unwittingly holding on to her emotional domain. In therapy with such couples I find that once this issue is addressed and the man obtains 'permission' from me and his wife to 'do intimate business' he soon makes great strides. It is amusing and instructive to see how such couples progress and how, on occasions, the woman becomes somewhat disquieted at her man's new-found abilities. Accepting that some males are actually better at various intimacy skills can be a real growth point, especially for the woman who was brought up to believe, consciously or unconsciously, that all men were a dead loss at this sort of thing.

We shall see on page 129 how to increase the amount of empathy in your relationship but here let us look at whether men *can* be empathic in a way that women want. The ability to put oneself into the shoes of others in order to be alongside them as they grapple with emotions is at the very heart of empathy. Most research has found that men are not nearly as good at this as women are. Things might not be quite this simple, however. Sophisticated studies have discovered that although males might not actually *display* such intimate connections, their level of physiological arousal, such as heart rate and blood pressure, is higher than that in females faced with similar emotional events. So it might simply be that women are good at externalizing by being empathic whereas men are better at internalizing. Clearly both types of behaviour have their advantages and disadvantages both for the individual and the relationship.

Perhaps, then, when a woman claims that her partner never listens to her and is unaffected by her emotions, his bodily 'knowledge' that this is untrue could be at the centre of many a disagreement over such matters. This kind of issue is often raised in discussions that have to do with gender difference on the subject of pain, sadness and bad news generally. Many men complain that their partner is a real 'tragedy queen', making a drama out of a minor matter, milking it for all it is worth, and so on. Women, on the other hand, say that their man simply does not see the problem. The truth appears to be that men are better at distracting themselves from such pain and do not ruminate upon it in the way that women do. Although many studies show that men are more out of touch with both their own feelings and those of others, this might not be all bad news if the alternative, as many see it, is to be constantly 'over-reacting to emotions, the way women do'.

Continued on page 74

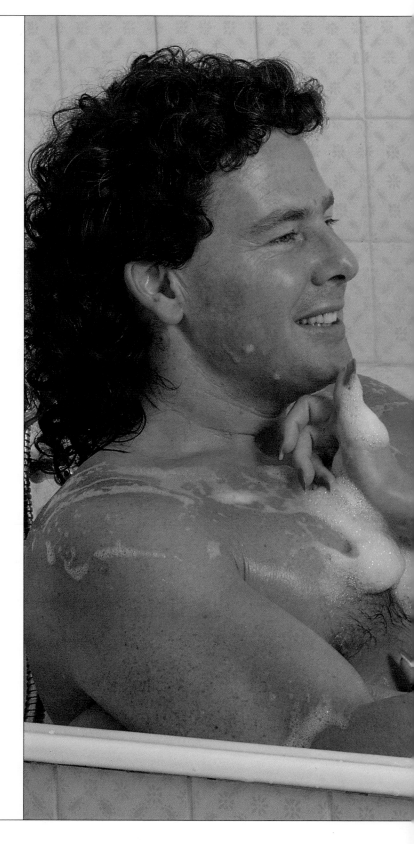

Adult games can have a similar significance to a father's paddling-pool fun with his young children (see page 68). Here he can learn to love, cherish and feel intimate with his partner without sex being on the agenda. After all, much of our loving life together as a couple is simply a reflection of joyous babyhood pleasures such as bathing, undressing, cuddling and feeling unconditionally loved.

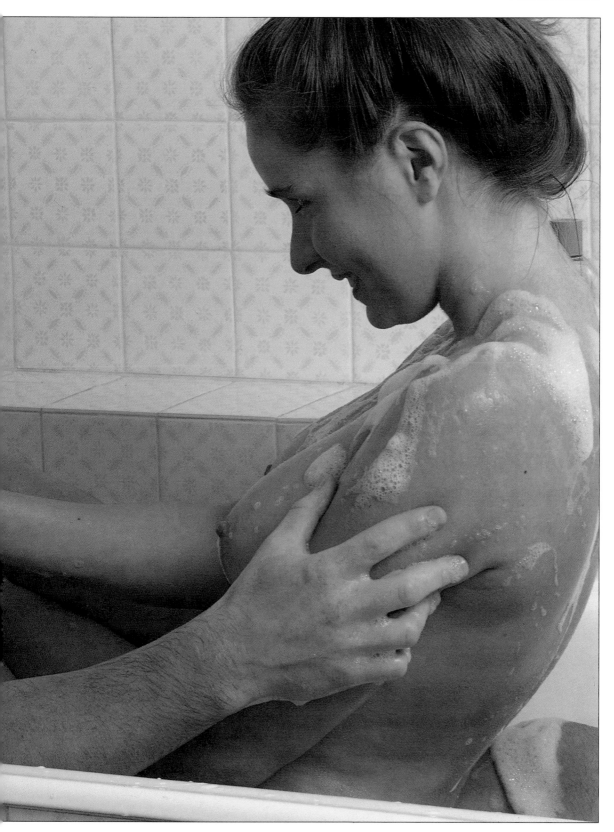

I try to look at this dispassionately with the couples I see, but it is indeed a fact that many women use huge amounts of energy dealing with their own emotions and those of others. All that can be said at the moment is that we simply do not know which of these gender-specific reactions is the more healthy overall. Perhaps, as with so many such issues, we need a balance of both types of behaviour between the sexes and within the sexes. The way men handle emotions might be just as 'right' as the way women do, at least in certain situations.

One of the commonest cries that I hear from women in the consulting room, in letters to me as an Agony Uncle and when I am running courses is that their man, and indeed men in general, cannot *express* their emotions. Women say that they are only too aware that their man is feeling *something* and that he often seems to know what it is, but that he cannot, or will not, name it, own it, or talk about it.

Although, generally speaking, it is true that men are less emotionally expressive than women, there are differences, depending upon the emotion being considered. Men tend, for example, to be less willing to express fear, sadness or negative emotions generally. Some of this is undoubtedly a reflection of the 'big boys don't cry' message that most males are reared with in our culture but there are other mechanisms at work too. It is interesting that this impoverished level of emotional expression, compared with women anyway, is mirrored in men's faces. Women show more emotion in their faces than men do, though there is no such difference among babies and very young children of both sexes. It appears that males become less expressive as a direct result of years of socialization.

Expressing emotions verbally is not, however, the only way that we show our conscious or unconscious underwear to others. Our body language tells others a lot too. It has been claimed that well over half of all human communication takes place at the non-verbal level so perhaps what we actually *say* is less important than what our body is telling the listener as we say it. One researcher found that non-verbal communication was about twice as powerful as what was being said.

When it comes to intimate communications men seem to be less able at using body language to sort out what is going on. For example, they are less good at recognizing how someone feels just by looking at the face; are less likely to maintain eye contact; keep a greater physical distance from others while talking to them; smile less; show fewer facial expressions generally, as we have seen; and use a voice style that is less conducive to sharing in an empathic way. Given that the vast majority of non-verbal communication is completely outside our conscious control, men will not be able to change many of these behaviour styles, except with considerable effort, and help from their partner. Once a man *is* aware of this sort of impediment to him becoming more intimate, though, things can be changed.

When men are talking they tend to dominate conversations; to talk to impress rather than to inform; to interrupt more; and to use verbal mastery to exert control. At the intensely personal level, however, the vast majority of men say that they greatly fear their partner's wrath on emotional issues because of her considerable superior verbal ability. This difference in behaviour within the private and public lives of couples has to be dealt with or it can be fatal flaw in the formation of an intimate relationship.

But who actually talk more, men or women? Many men say that women talk too much, yet studies repeatedly find that it is men who talk most, whether it is at meetings, mixed-sex discussions or in classrooms. Men also usually speak for longer once they start. In one study the women's longest bouts of speaking were shorter than the men's shortest ones. At professional meetings, or indeed any meetings where men and women come together to have a say, men's comments from the audience are always longer than women's and they ask more questions and make more comments than the women present do.

In public, then, men talk more, probably because they feel more comfortable with it. In private, though, the polarity is reversed, with women saying more. This probably comes about as men, so ready to impress and inform in public, realize that in private their partners are looking for something else: 'talk' that enables connection and deals with emotions. For most men talk establishes status and preserves independence whereas for most women it is a way of creating and maintaining connections and networks.

Let us now look at whether men might *need* intimacy less than women do. It could, after all, be that men are less good at intimacy because they do not need it. Certainly if you ask a group of people what they think about this most women say that their need for intimacy is great and that their man's need is little. In fact, most women claim that emotional sharing is central to a 'real' relationship and that they value a man who can do this kind of emotional business. If we look at all the studies done on the subject since the Second World War the majority have found that women put 'poor communication' at the top of their list of reasons for divorce or separation. Men do not perceive it to be nearly as important and some see it as totally unimportant.

If studies from all over the world are compared it is clear that men everywhere fear intimacy as defined by women to some extent. Two studies have found that males link thoughts of danger and violence with scenes of affiliation and intimacy. This could partly explain a well-recognized behavioural trait that men exhibit when faced with an emotional threat. They project their own fears and internal woundedness on to others by using blaming or attacking behaviour whereas women tend to internalize their emotions and blame themselves. This sort of thinking has led to the commonly quoted male assertion that 'A woman's place is in the wrong'. Indeed clinical experience in almost any sort of relationship work shows that the average Western woman can easily be made to feel guilty about almost anything. This is nothing short of tragic and has fateful implications for man-woman relationships. Interestingly, a recent study found that women over forty feared intimacy more than men of the same age did and that females seemed to rate intimacy less as they aged.

It is perhaps because of men's fear of their unconscious reflex reaction to act out or externalize inner emotional pains that they tend to withdraw, become socially isolated or to suppress painful feelings by using work, drugs or alcohol. This removes them from the potential healing available from their partner's willingness to be intimate. Many men tell me, however, that they do not see this so much as a healing opportunity lost but self-preservatory behaviour that removes them from yet further hurt. It could be that they feel unable to deal with the magnitude of their own emotions and then project this sense of helplessness and hopelessness on to their partner who, according to the man's unconscious, would not be able to deal with them either. If the emotions are too big for either or both of them to cope with, his unconscious continues, he would be better off going away and 'dealing with them' on his own somehow.

Most women I see with a partner like this are at the same time telling their sons, usually quite unconsciously it is true, that they should suppress their emotions, be strong, not cry, not be 'like a girl' or whatever. Small wonder then that the average adult male believes that the emotional arena is somehow littered with the corpses of those who even dare to deal with such matters. They were well trained by females to believe it.

But does all this matter? Do men suffer in any way as a result of their relative inability to be intimate? Research has found that people who are able to be intimate are better at coping with life's stressful events. Several experts have wondered whether men's earlier age of death compared with women might have something to do with their relatively poor intimacy skills. It could be that men suffer because they have few social support structures compared with women and that this, coupled with their poor ability to express feelings, might bring about stress illnesses. Certainly it is well proven that people who have good social supports fare better in the hurly-burly of life than those who do not. One study found that having a significant, close person protected against ill health to some extent. An Israeli study found that men who did not have such a person were more likely to have a heart attack than were other comparable males.

It has long been known that men's health fares exceptionally badly after the loss of an intimate partner. Recent studies looking at suicide, mental illness and death rates highlight the considerable significance of a love-bonded partner to the average male. Marriage in particular suits men very well and they do rather badly on the loss of it. Women, on the other hand, are more likely to be mentally ill if they are married rather than single. So clearly a love-bonded relationship, even if it is not intimate by many women's definition, is very valuable to the average man.

Males also seem to be heavily dependent on their relationship with their significant female. Given that this is usually the only intimate or near-intimate relationship that they have, the loss of it is greatly feared in advance and brings considerable problems for most when it happens. Women, on the other hand, have many more such intimate bonds and so miss their partner less from this point of view. Also, as women age they form even greater networks of significant people with whom they can be intimate, whereas research shows that men become more isolated and dependent on their one-to-one relationship as the years go by. If couples are asked to rate their views separately about intimacy, more women say they are wary of disclosing their personal feelings to their husbands than the other way around and more husbands claim to feel understood by their wives than the reverse. Looked at as a whole, therefore, men get a better deal when it comes to intimacy yet stand to lose far more because they have all their eggs in one basket.

Some studies have found that repeated suppression of how we feel can damage our health. There is little doubt that the ways in which many men cope with the discomfort of emotions (work, drinking, smoking, gambling, over-eating and so on) can be injurious in themselves. In fact the more macho the man in terms of emotional suppression, the more likely he is to suffer from stress diseases and to be generally ill.

Many men say that they would rather not become over-involved in emotions because it seems to cost their female friends and acquaintances so dearly. After all, they argue, are not many more women mentally ill than men? Recent reassessments of old statistics suggest that this is a foolish way to look at the subject. Women do not have more mental and emotional illness overall, as was previously claimed. To make a realistic comparison between the sexes, one has to be aware of all the alcoholism, substance abuse, criminality and self-destructive sexual behaviour so commonly indulged in by men and add these to the list of commonly accepted male mental illnesses. Here again we see women internalizing the blame whilst externalizing the emotions while men act out their emotional pain by 'doing' (suicide, violence and crime generally) or 'avoiding' (social isolation, alcoholism and drug abuse).

What, then, can be concluded from all this evidence about men and intimacy? On the one hand is the view that males are largely socialized in a way that discourages the expression of emotions. The solution, according to this theory, is to alter the way that boys are reared so that they are more able to express their emotions, be more empathic, more expressive generally and better able to use body language as a way of encoding and decoding emotions. We saw on page 28 that female-only parenting also has a profound effect on later outcomes. On the other hand there are those who argue that males and females are different at a fundamental biological level. They think and behave differently right from birth, for example, and that these differences persist no matter how we bring children up. Here, as with many similar issues, the old nature versus nurture dichotomy persists and looks like doing so for some time.

To a large extent, though, it hardly matters who is right because, as in so many such matters, there is no totally 'right' answer. Both male and female models of intimacy have their advantages and disadvantages. Men would certainly benefit from expressing themselves better and by being more open; and women would benefit from being more assertive and taking more power and control. Women's greater reliance on others is a somewhat double-edged sword; men's desire to remain self-reliant and based in the 'certainty' of the material world leaves them wide open to isolation and loneliness while defending them against many of the ills that women's attention to the emotional needs of others brings upon them.

As I have mentioned elsewhere, we have become used to thinking that our partner should provide us with all that we need from a one-to-one relationship. But even assuming that our perceptions of what we need are correct, and very often they are not, it is unwise to look to our partner to be everything for us. Women are probably going to feel short-changed in the world of intimacy for the foreseeable future as men strive to catch up on various skills that could help both parties. In the meantime women will have to look elsewhere for the sort of intimate relation-

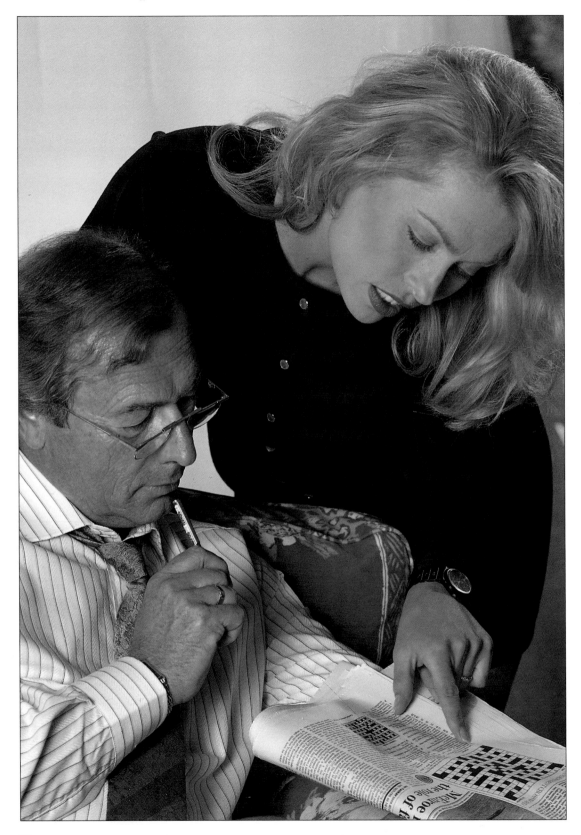

ships they want or need. Women can usually find this fairly easily in the company of other women but for the man who finds his partner unable to be intimate the situation is more dangerous. Such a man understandably looks to another woman to fill the gap but she all too often perceives this to be the start of a sexual relationship. It is still rare in our culture for men and women to be intimate friends and yet be sexually inactive. Perhaps this is just one of many areas of social life that will change for the better as more of us become able to be truly intimate and to separate intimacy from sex.

Before leaving the battle of the sexes it is perhaps interesting to point out that many women claim that they feel more put down by other females than by men. This is a vast subject that cannot adequately be dealt with here, but suffice it to say that many a woman uses her intimacy skills to the disadvantage of her fellow females, both consciously and unwittingly. Some of the reasons for this were examined on page 28. Another interesting angle is that considerable numbers of women have told me that many females are not all that able at being intimate. I often hear this in respect of my patients' mothers. Similarly, both sexes frequently claim that their father was much more empathic or able to be intimate than their mother ever was. Indeed I have had many female patients over the years who have had little or no success with female therapists but have done very well with me, a male, with whom they found they could 'do intimate business' much more easily than with another female. Whether we are thinking about the gender of a therapist or about our partner it is helpful to remember that the feminine component in any man and the masculine in any woman can hugely alter the entire picture. This paradox means that there are men who are much more capable of empathy and intimacy from their loving, nurturing, feminine parts than are many women. It is also true that many women are more forceful, goal-centred and driven than some men. And all of these forces change and rebalance as a relationship matures.

The picture is therefore complex and easily hijacked by stereotypical thinking. It behoves us all to bear this in mind no matter what sort of relationship we are engaged in at work, home or play. There is no doubt in my mind that any couple's journey towards greater intimacy must address the gender differences they perceive between them. Few couples who persist in the stereotypical model of the 'all-feeling female' and the 'emotionally crippled male' ever get anywhere. We shall probably never know whether women are 'too emotional' and rely 'too much' on intimacy; or whether men are somehow 'deficient' in these areas of life. It should not greatly matter to any couple determined to grow together in their intimate life. Both can learn from the other. This shared experience of learning together could well make redundant all the theories about who is 'right'.

Simply doing everyday things together can reinforce true intimacy in a relationship. This is the real intimacy 'foreplay' that makes subsequent bedroom sex rewarding. Even something as simple as helping with the crossword can create an atmosphere of mutual support that reverberates throughout the relationship.

'KNOWING' AND BEING RIGHT

There are few more powerful barriers to creating an intimate life than 'being right'. We all believe that we are 'normal', so we tend to think that what we 'know', believe or think is somehow right. This means that when we come across others who differ from us their views are immediately somehow 'wrong', if only by our definition. This process creates a kind of play in which we are not only the central actor but also the producer and script-writer. When we try to deal with our partner he or she comes into the play as a sort of guest actor and is supposed to read from our script and act according to our direction.

It is easy to see, once I use this analogy, how hopeless this can make the 'guest actor' feel who has little or no control over his or her part in the play or its outcome. This righteousness (a certainty that we are right from our own point of view) bedevils almost all one-to-one relationships, and to those that involve close partners who are trying to be intimate it is a real killer.

For an individual trapped in this sort of behaviour pattern it is often more important to be right or to 'know' than it is to love or be loved. I have had countless experiences of people, often men, who would rather throw up their whole relationship than admit that their world-view or personal belief structure could be 'wrong'. There is no such thing as right or wrong on the vast majority of occasions yet it can be very hard to sell this idea to most people. The thought that directly opposing views might *both* be right in their own way is a difficult or impossible nettle for many of us to grasp. It appears to strike at the heart of our certainty, our very being.

One of the areas of life that is most plagued by such righteousness is the sexual arena we share with our partner. As we try to be faithful in a one-to-one relationship we have few opportunities to test our feelings or rightness or 'knowing' with others; therefore we do not have the same opportunity that we would in other spheres of life to feel our way and alter our views. Monogamous relationships reduce our opportunities to learn and modify our deeply held convictions, let alone to rewrite our script.

Although this applies to many areas of life together, it is in matters to do with sex that we are most trapped by our expectations, by our original script which, we then assert, must be adhered to by our partner if he or she wishes to deal with us. Unfortunately this defensive posture is self-destructive. It leaves us isolated and lonely as we discover that others also have their scripts and want to direct their own play. The scene is now set for conflict as the individual tells me that he would rather be right than 'give in' to his partner. People who insist on being sure 'know' what is true or, as I say to pull their leg, they 'seem to have a direct line to God' on the matter under consideration. This 'knowing' usually extends to knowing far more about the other than about themselves, yet for all this knowledge they remain unloved, unloving and unlovable.

The business of knowing about our partner in this way is an enemy of intimacy. It shuts out the reality of what and who our partner is unless this happens to fall within the definitions we have laid down. Such 'knowing' or being right also prevents us from really knowing ourselves because we are too busy reading the script and directing the players. Very few people in this situation actually consider rewriting the script as, after all, it is already 'right', by definition.

The saddest part about 'knowing' is that it prevents us from growing. Being sure that what we know is the final word on the subject not only stops us being intimate by shutting out others and their truths, but it also blocks our own change and learning. I always claim, when teaching on this issue, that most experience is spurious. This usually brings forth considerable anger or an even worse reaction because most people, especially those who consider themselves to be 'experienced' in whatever field we are discussing, think that they have gained hugely from it. My contention is that most of us learn rather little from experience, except how to do things in much the same way we always have. But this is not growing and changing. Having done something the same inappropriate or wrong way for forty years does not make us 'experienced', except perhaps at repeatedly making the same mistake.

Real experience that can be claimed to be useful comes from being sufficiently mature to be open to change and learning. This is nowhere to be seen more piquantly than in the sexual life. Men, especially, claim that because they have had several partners before they married (or after for that matter) 'know' what women want or need. Their current partner is climbing the wall because he cannot or will not supply what *she* needs and his adherence to his rightness often makes her feel angry. This same process can take place in exactly the same way in emotional matters between a couple.

Such a man may well be 'sure' and 'experienced' but he is also lonely and miserable because he cannot connect with his lover. Such an individual also has very little fun. To be open enough to play and have fun we have to accept that we might be 'wrong' rather than have all the answers. This playfulness eludes millions of couples because they are unconsciously loath to return to the childlike state of unknowing that makes play and pleasure possible and rewarding.

The profound truth behind all this is that how we see matters is not how they actually are but simply how they appear to us to be. The Mayan Indians had a wonderful saying, 'All life is an illusion', and how right they were. Almost anything viewed from a different angle can appear very different, yet all those seeing it are right in their perception of it. When we start to believe that what we 'see' is real, as opposed to our particular illusion, we get into trouble. So it is that our 'knowledge' on most things, rather than freeing us to be ourselves, traps us, and often our partner too. Intimacy as I define it clearly cannot thrive in such a setting. Even knowing ourselves is a lifetime's task, let alone knowing our partner. Only foolhardy individuals would make the claim that they know their partner better than they know themselves.

It is only when we are intimate that we can 'know'. We touch our real selves by contacting them in the presence of another. This 'reality' is now rooted in our experience of ourselves in our partner's presence. This is the only learning worthy of the name. When I do this I am alone in the presence of my partner doing *my* business, not hers. This is usually confused with being lonely but the two are very different. We all come into the world alone and leave it alone. The journey to greater intimacy is essentially a task we carry out alone, albeit in the presence of our loved one. This is very different from being lonely, with all the negative emotions that this brings. Our partner cannot teach us to be intimate; he or she cannot make us feel intimate either. What our partner can do is to be himself or herself while we discover about ourselves. This means accepting that we are not 'right'; that we do not 'know'; that we are simply using our connection with our partner to trudge on our own personal journey towards intimacy.

It is a tragedy that all of this becomes more dangerous as we live together for many years. 'I know exactly what he's going to say', is what some people say to me about their partner in our sessions. I often challenge such a remark by saying that I have no idea what he is going to say and then ask him to speak, after first getting the 'sure' individual to write down what he or she thinks is coming next. This partner is often surprised, largely, to be fair, because the individual who is talking feels sufficiently free to be himself or herself in the presence of an impartial third party. For a moment, the partner's script is thrown out and the speaker refuses to act in the play.

Such 'already knowing' really wreaks havoc in bed too. Once we become certain about our partner's sexuality we are limited by this 'illusion' and ironically limit his or her growth. Many's the time I hear the replay of an affair while I watch the gaping mouth of the partner who cannot believe what he or she is hearing. This is not the partner he or she 'knows'. How could their partner possibly behave in such a way? This sort of conversation gives us the opportunity to discover just how boring and repetitive their sex life has become and how their both being 'right' about one another or themselves has limited their passion and their creativity. Many people say that it is the 'not knowing' that makes extra-marital sex such fun and so passionate. I think this speaks for itself.

RAISING CHILDREN WHO CAN BE INTIMATE

Whenever I speak publicly about intimacy the commonest question that people, especially women, raise is, 'How can I bring up my children, particularly my boys, so that they will be more able to be intimate when they are adults?' There are no easy answers to this (though I explore some provocatively fundamental possibilities on page 28). It is fairly obvious, however, that our children learn about most things directly from us, their parents, usually at a somewhat unconscious-to-unconscious level. This is perhaps more true of intimacy than many other matters because much of the very essence of intimacy is rather intangible and cannot be directly taught to children. Intimacy is, *par excellence*, a behaviour and 'being' style that children absorb with the air they breathe in a home where intimacy is commonplace between adults.

We can also learn a great deal about intimacy *from* our children, however. Many people say that one of the best things about being a parent is that their children teach them so much. Young, pre-school children in particular can give their parents a jewel-like window on intimacy that is unaffected by the world outside. Few of us who are parents can deny that our children have made us more aware of our humanness, our weaknesses and our imperfections. This in itself is a priceless gift towards our intimate life-style as a couple. In fact many parents claim that their children forced them to learn about themselves in a way that would not, and indeed did not happen, when they were child-free.

The business of bringing up children gives adults something creative to do as a team: a goal to strive for that is essentially selfless. This can also help with the adults' personal growth and their intimate life as a couple. When trying to sort out differences between us as parents so that we can present a united front to our children we learn how to make adjustments; how to do deals; and how to compromise. We also have to start accepting how different our children are both from us as their parents and from the other youngsters in the family. Having said this, one of the most painful challenges in this area is to confront the *similarities* between ourselves and our children. Seeing our worst traits in others so young can sometimes force us to change our own attitudes and behaviour. This process of self-examination and personal growth forces most parents to grow up and mature in a way that they might otherwise not have done; and this change means that the parents themselves become more able to be intimate with one another.

So much for the positive side. Now for the problems. Families, because they are by definition 'familiar' and 'close', can hamper the development of true intimacy. Most of us try to maintain a considerable degree of closeness in our family. Historically, people have always tried to keep their family together; in doing so, however, they created a sort of 'system' made up of individuals whose main task was to further the future of that system. Family therapists the world over look at such systems when things are going wrong in families. In such families in one sense, however, *any* sort of system harms intimacy because if we are constantly trying to put the formation and maintenance of relationships above the process of discovering our true selves, intimacy will always suffer.

In every family, then, there is a tension between the members being 'close' in order to maintain relationships and each individual trying to discover his or her identity in a personal quest for intimacy. Perhaps it is now possible to see the difficulties involved in actively encouraging children to be intimate. By doing so it can at first appear that the relationships within the family might suffer or even that family integrity itself will be harmed. Yet successful families that raise children to be autonomous adults who can be intimate with others carefully balance these two apparently conflicting systems. There is enough closeness for relationships to flourish yet enough autonomy and individuality for personal discovery and growth to lead to the capacity for intimacy.

Parents who work through this book and enrich their intimate life together will certainly get more pleasure from their family life; will be more effective as parents; and will discover roads into their own unconscious that would be difficult to find in any other way. Children not only make us face ourselves in a manner that few other situations can but also give us an opportunity to build a more intimate world as our example rubs off on them. This multiplier effect of intimate parenting is perhaps one hope for the future of family life at a time when the omens are not very rosy. In this sense the smaller families of today probably help us all. Many older people have told me how difficult it was trying to be intimate with large numbers of children. There should be some intimacy advantages to having only two children.

INTIMACY AND SPIRITUALITY

When asked, the vast majority of people claim that they believe in some sort of 'God' or supernatural creator being. Most people I deal with also say that they know that there is a side to themselves, and indeed all humans, that transcends the mere flesh and blood that makes up their physical bodies. Once we try to advance on this front, though, matters start to become more confused as each one of us has our own ideas and experiences of what the 'spiritual' world means to us.

Most people in our largely secular culture find it difficult at first to talk of spirituality without being side-tracked by issues to do with religion. Indeed most people with whom I discuss the subject imagine that I am referring to religion when in fact I am not. There are few people who are without an experience of their transcendent self whether it be in sex; when painting a picture; playing an instrument; praying; communing with nature; or whatever. In such pursuits we exceed our mechanical body and our trained mind and elevate ourselves to another plane. In this we find a new self, or probably more accurately, our true self that normal everyday life masks from us.

One of the reasons that intimacy is so difficult to define is that it is not just a learned *behaviour* but also a spiritual *experience*. How can we adequately describe, explain, or rationalize the magical effect of a painting, a landscape, a musical phrase, a colour, or whatever that we discover takes us into our spiritual world? So it is with intimacy with other human beings.

Intimacy, then, is largely a spiritual experience. It can be an emotional and physical one too, but at its core it takes us out of our mind and body into another world in which we connect with nature in all its forms, not just with the individual with whom we are being intimate at that time.

As we saw earlier, some people claim to be more intimate with nature or even with inanimate objects than they are with people. At one extreme this can be the sign of severe mental disturbance, but in moderation it is not in itself harmful. A patient of mine was able to communicate better with inanimate objects than with the people around about him and his skill at this made him a gifted artist. It was ironic to many who knew him that he was more able to be intimate in his special way than most of those who claimed to be so in their personal relationships. He was able to be truly himself in the presence of the subject he was painting, while it was being truly itself. This honesty and integrity led him to artistic expressions of his spirituality that were impossible for him to experience in human relationships. Ironically, his art communicated his core being to people with an intimacy that was not possible in what most people would call normal human relationships. He touched their soul indirectly through the medium of his art.

Today's materialistic world is characterized by people becoming increasingly isolated from their environment and from those around them, yet it appears that humans crave connection with these very things. When we are intimate with another person we sense this in our innermost parts and for that moment share in the miracle of life and our own humanness. When we transcend our bodily being and become truly intimate we yield; and through this giving up we contact shared automony. This, for many, is an experience they call spiritual.

This is where sex starts to fit into the whole context of intimacy. Sex as a physical union of two people takes place at the bodily level, but there are few who would claim that the sort of sex that means most to them stops here. The spiritual nature of sexual intercourse and everything that surrounds it is all too real to most people, even if they have never expressed it openly to anyone. Sex is perfectly possible without intimacy but sex *with* intimacy becomes something very different. As we shall see later it is this craving for transcendent spiritual experience that makes sex such a sought-after commodity today. To many it has become a kind of religion and it is easy to see why.

FORGIVENESS

In the in-tray on my filing cabinet I have a small piece of paper that has sat there for many years. On it I wrote a long time ago, 'He who cannot forgive breaks the bridge over which he himself must pass.' Every week as I file my notes and papers I come across this reminder to be more forgiving in my work and my personal life.

Very little is said about forgiveness today. Indeed I have read countless books and learned papers about marriage and relationships over the years and the subject is rarely mentioned. Yet at the heart of any intimate relationship must lie the ability to forgive both ourselves and our partner. It is often said that we should 'forgive and forget', but I believe the sign of real maturity is to forgive and *remember*. When we forgive we do not deny or avoid what has happened, and we do not wipe the slate clean, yet we forgive. How can we do this and be true to ourselves?

In our one-to-one relationships we all create and experience indifference, rejection, unloving behaviour, humiliation, discourtesy, disrespect, and much more, yet somehow we have to go on with life, preferably without bearing grudges. Few of us go around deliberately creating hell for others. When we find ourselves at fault we quickly realize what we have done and feel remorse, sorrow, sadness, guilt or something similar. It is usually easiest to forgive people if we believe that they are sorry and that they will try not to do the same again.

In an intimate relationship, or one that is striving to become intimate, we really have no choice but to forgive one another. The burden of carrying the anger, frustration or whatever is so great that it kills the very thing we are trying to create. Furthermore, as with so many of these relationship paradoxes, the individual who does *not* forgive is often the one who suffers more as a result. Such unresolved emotions become a sort of personal prison for ourselves, while our partner, the original and apparent source of the pain, is relatively unharmed. In my experience, both personally and professionally, the tiniest remnant of unforgiven business can poison the rest of the relationship.

If I feel wounded because someone has hurt me, only I can heal my wounds. The only way I know of doing this is to forgive the other person. To do anything else is to hurt myself more and this is perverse. When reading this, some might think 'What a saint he must be', but exactly the reverse is true. It is only by being aware that we need the forgiveness of others and ourselves, if we are to stand a chance of intimacy, that we can hope truly to forgive others. In this sense, if I forgive you, I help myself; and if I forgive myself, I help us.

Problems arise when the one we love hurts or abuses us on an ongoing basis in some way, such as with physical attacks, drug addiction, bad language, attacking behaviour, refusal of sex, anger or withdrawal; the list is enormous. Only a masochistic personality will seek to perpetuate such abuse and most of us do not tolerate it. We can, however, still forgive while we are putting an end to the abuse. If an individual has a need, however unconscious, to continue to inflict pain – physical or emotional – on his or her partner, then the relationship is dead. We have a duty to protect ourselves from those who hurt us repeatedly, even if they appear not to do so intentionally. Making the decision to call it a day after having forgiven time and again can be very difficult and is one that I frequently work on with couples. Women, particularly, often continue with their relationship in the hope of rescuing their man from himself, healing him or somehow 'winning', but the whole relationship degenerates into a sort of ongoing battle rather than one in which forgiveness occurs in parallel with getting away from the source of the pain.

I get such couples to agree to a deadline for the end of the abusive behaviour. This gives the one on the receiving end some hope that life will not be intolerable for ever; gives the alcoholic/drug-abuser/wife-beater/child-abuser/workaholic a chance to mend his or her ways in therapy; and enables us all to create sufficient goodwill to break old attitudes and patterns. Set against this background, real forgiveness is often possible. The abuser and the abused can work together to learn how to stop the pernicious dance of death in which they are playing their respective roles.

Perhaps the best thing about forgiving a partner is the wonderful clean feeling we get as we let go of the hurt. It frees us to get on with life again. Having said this, how do we actually make it happen? First of all we need to look into ourselves and try to discover why we were so hurt by what our partner did. Think of your inner shadow (see page 35). If the event was a one-off then things are often fairly simple but if it was part of an ongoing pattern we need to change our attitudes as does our partner. Such changes will then usually lead to alterations in behaviour.

Once we can be open with our mate and truly forgive or be forgiven we should be able to put the issue away and agree not to bring it up again. This calls for courage and many of us are simply not that brave. When we put the issue away we really have to *believe* that it is gone, not, as I often find, pretend to ourselves that it is but keep on vigilantly watching just in case, like a prowler in the night, it actually has not. I often ask people if they are big enough to forgive their mate. This is a challenge most people would like to meet. Many soon realize, however, that they cannot, and need to grow within themselves before they are able to find the courage, the inner warrior, to be able to forgive. Even more courage is called for when we find ourselves needing to be forgiven. Most of us find it easier to give than receive and easier to forgive than be forgiven.

She has just told him of an affair she had last year. He knows that
he has to forgive her if they are to survive and grow as a couple. Not to
forgive means that he will suffer more than she. Such generosity of spirit
is at the very heart of intimate relationships.

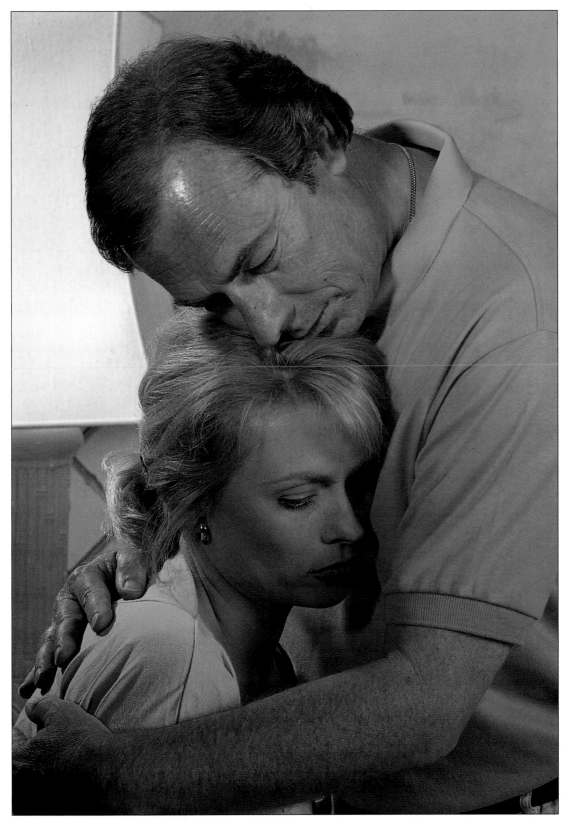

Our Judaeo-Christian society often gives us the impression that if we wrong someone we must perform some sort of penance or be punished. It is sad when this is the case in one-to-one relationships because in a loving union no one has to be punished in order to be forgiven. Being separated from our beloved at a spiritual level is punishment enough. If we are forgiven no punishment is needed and we should try hard not to punish ourselves. Time and again I see women who punish themselves by having all their hair cut off (or something similar) after having transgressed within their sexual relationship. Their partner may have truly forgiven them yet they continue to chastise themselves, in this case by sadistically removing one of the manifestations of their 'tarty behaviour'. They are not consciously aware at the time that this is what they are doing, but often spontaneously offer such an explanation at a later date.

Perhaps most difficult for the one who is forgiven is to accept that forgiving and being forgiven is not some sort of business deal. If you forgive me I do not have to prove that I am worthy of it or deserve it. You freely forgive me and that is all there is to it. I cannot earn your forgiveness. In a culture that encourages deals of all kinds this 'free gift' approach comes as a surprise or is seen as suspect. Many people who consult me have problems with such no-strings-attached situations and believe that at some time they will *have* to pay. This is no basis for intimacy.

Lastly, a real problem for many people is learning to forgive themselves. We are very tough on ourselves in Western society and, believing that we are unworthy of forgiveness, unconsciously project this on to our partner as if he or she were too. Such lack of self-love cripples us and prevents us from truly loving our partner. Growth stops both within ourselves and within the relationship.

None of this subject will be easy to deal with if it is fresh ground for you. If this is the case turn to page 155 where there are some exercises to help you practise how to forgive and be forgiven.

KNOW THYSELF

Given that so many of us are aware of the Ancient Greek saying, 'First know thyself', it is perhaps surprising that Western concepts of 'self' are so poor. When psychologists or philosophers do write about it, it is usually seen as some sort of mystical, Eastern or philosophical concept. Indeed, many people have little or no concrete notion of what their self is. To many it is most closely allied to the concept of the soul, the very essence of a person. Notions of 'I' or 'me' are not nearly as central to our being as is our sense of self. I can usually say what *I* am. You can tell me what you think of *me*. But how do we deal with one another's *selves*?

Our deepest nature, this self, can make itself known through dreams, creativity, non-verbal communication, religious and mystical experiences and many other areas of life from which the 'I' and the 'me' are largely excluded. Jung claimed that the self was indescribable and most learned thinkers deal with it only in terms of idiom and metaphysics. Yet for all this we appear to learn about our sense of self from those around us very early in life, and possibly even in the womb.

I can know who 'I' am in relation to you; I can experience 'me' when I am in my own space; but to know my 'self' I have to share a space with creation at the intimate level. It is possible and arguably desirable to modify our 'I' experience in order to enhance our total experience with someone who is 'other' than us. This is neither passive nor negative but is done out of healthy self-centredness, of which more in a moment.

It is essential to be open to change if we are to enjoy real intimacy, yet many couples are somewhat conditional about change. They say something like, '*I* am prepared to change but first *you* will have to do some changing'. Such a couple have lost touch, if they ever had it, with their personal power to take responsibility for their 'selves' in their relationship.

We all owe it to ourselves to try to discover as much as we can about the real self within. This is one of our famous paradoxes because just about the best way of discovering about our selves is by being intimate with the creation. I use this rather pompous word because it is not enough simply to strive for intimacy with our nearest and dearest. Our partner is only one source of intimacy. We could well learn more about our real self from 'being' with a daffodil, or touching the sand on the sea-shore than we could with our partner at a particular time. This connectedness with nature, animate and inanimate, is all part of our journey towards greater intimacy with our beloved.

This might sound somewhat mystical or even weird to many readers, but in others it will strike a real chord. I often see people who are almost totally at odds with their innermost selves and yet expect to enjoy a meaningful relationship with their partner, their children or whomever. Others are almost entirely disconnected from their environment and find it difficult to understand why intimacy seems to elude them in their human relationships.

During therapy with such individuals, it is never long before they raise the issue of selfishness implicit in the pursuit of increased 'self'-knowledge and respect. We live in a somewhat Christian culture in which it is wrongly assumed that Jesus commanded us to 'love our neighbour *more* than ourselves'. In fact he said that we were to 'love our neighbour *as* ourselves' – in the same way that we love ourselves. Many people soon realize that they love themselves very little and so have no well of love from which to draw in order to nurture others. Yet before we embark on such a discussion in therapy, most such folk claim to be very loving. The implausibility of the original situation soon becomes apparent, however, as they begin really to love themselves. Notions of the greater importance of others are so deeply embedded in our culture that the journey to get people to focus on themselves rather than others is often a long one. Many fight me tooth and nail as I insist that they stop doing things to and for others until they can be sure that what they are doing is coming from the right place: their core self. Anything other than this is an elegant, if unconscious, way of duping our partner and all those around us.

So how can we hope to know ourselves? First we can open ourselves up to opportunities to connect with nature in its many forms. Next, we can start on a journey that allows us to believe that we might be wrong about many things (see page 80); and by allowing ourselves to be wrong, we discover what it is about ourselves that made us so certain.

Thirdly, we can use our partner to help us grow into greater intimacy. This will

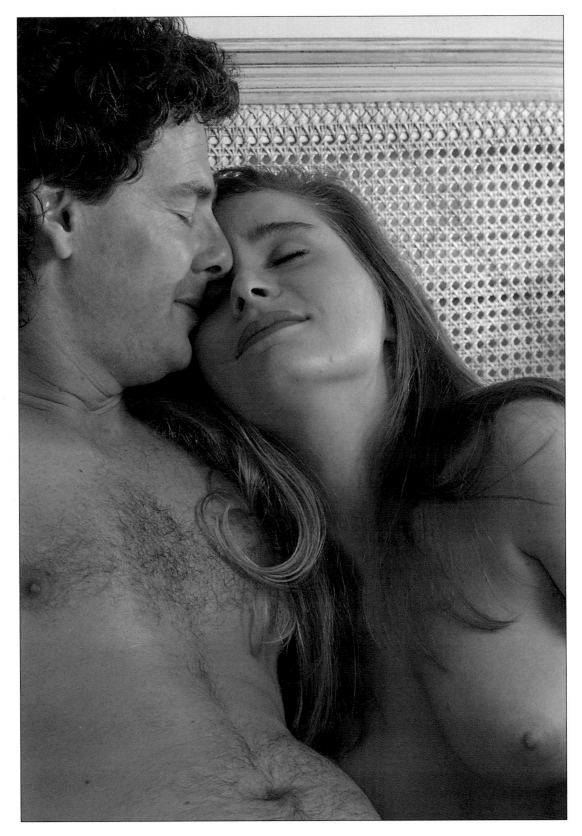

enable us to be truly ourselves in his or her presence, loved unconditionally and valid for ourselves, just as we are. In this state it is possible to touch depths of self-hood that are impossible to grasp in any other way. This soul-to-soul connection allows us safely to reflect our core being off another in a way that we never have previously experienced. The fortunate individual will be familiar with this from their childhood and babyhood but many I meet have never known this kind of soul-to-soul touching and are very frightened of it. They do not know their real selves; fear that because they do not, that it is somehow unknowable; and that last time they tried to be truly known in this way (in the cradle) they failed to touch and be touched at this core level and do not want to fail again. Yet it is only by risking another failure that we stand any chance of ever knowing our real selves. Such risk-taking is the only route to a touching of souls with our partner.

All of this is far being from selfish in the Christian, pejorative sense of the word; it is highly selfless because by really coming to know our '*self*' we allow others to be themselves, unique creations in the universe. This is where intimacy begins.

We shall see on page 98 how important all this is for better sex. I see many couples who feel closest and what they call intimate during sex. Yet once they start to become truly intimate, knowing and valuing themselves as unique creations, their sexual life blossoms in ways that they never thought possible. Sex now becomes a somewhat mystical and spiritual experience, albeit firmly rooted in the pleasures and rewards of the here-and-now. Such couples have little trouble remaining faithful to one another over long periods of time because they do not have sex with their genitals alone but with their whole core being.

In the final analysis, therefore, if we are to learn about intimacy we first have to learn about ourselves, warts and all. Constantly looking at the other person and not ourselves gets us nowhere. As I often say to my patients, 'Start off by turning the spotlight inwards. Open us a few boxes in the cellar and get out the things that have not seen the light of day. When you have sorted all these out, we will start to look at how and what your partner should change.' This task takes a lifetime, but the journey itself takes us into a self-knowledge that benefits everyone we know, especially our partner.

THE COST OF INTIMACY

Most people who claim to want a more intimate life say that they would 'do anything' to make it happen. Once we start to talk about the responsibilities of intimacy, however – the commitment required, the effort and time involved – many start to think again. This is hardly surprising given that the rewards for the effort put into intimacy often go unnoticed by others and sometimes even by ourselves.

Try to make special times for one another to recapture those moments when you felt really loved and intimate. Most of us are so busy that we put a low priority on such intimacies and then wonder why we lose touch with one another. The answer is in our own hands.

So what are the costs likely to be? First of all, building a more intimate life definitely takes time. This can be a lot more difficult than we think. The average couple spends less than twenty minutes a day dealing with one another at any one-to-one level, let alone being truly intimate. The astonishing fact is that we spend far longer with others in our lives than we do with our partner. Over the years, especially if we have a family, the time we spend together decreases year by year until the children leave home, which is when things can improve for many.

Making a special time for yourselves every week and then additionally creating little breaks when you can get away from the routine of life together are the surest ways of enabling yourselves to become more intimate. I have yet to find a couple who rarely spend time with one another and yet are intimate. It is not a matter of saying 'We're intimate and that's it'. Most of us find that our intimate life needs servicing, and this takes time.

The next cost that is worth thinking about is energy. It is never easy taking an existing relationship onwards towards change and growth. Even if you can readily make the time there is still a formidable cost in energy if you intend to move matters on. Our old attitudes, our 'knowing' what is right and much other unconscious baggage takes a lot of energy to shift or throw out. Just one of the simplest exercises in Part Three of this book could leave you feeling exhausted for days, such is the effort required. Much of the work involved in creating an intimate life means breaking down old defences. This in itself is hard emotional work. Given that our unconscious tries to erect new defences to protect itself, the construction gang cannot go off duty either. So early on in the task both work-forces are flat out, respectively building and demolishing defences, often at the same time. This is hard work and can only be done at the rate at which any one individual can cope with it.

There may also be a financial cost involved in building intimacy. Things will have to change as you shift your relationship towards greater intimacy. Some of these might cost money. It could be, for example, that you decide to work fewer hours in the week; not to work at weekends; to make more time for yourselves away from home together; to have holidays; to buy books about relationship issues; perhaps to go into therapy to resolve issues that arise; and so on.

I have yet to meet a couple who found their journey towards greater intimacy all plain sailing. Another cost worth knowing about early on is the pain you will almost certainly experience as you give up old ways of thinking, being and behaving. These old systems do not just disappear peacefully in our sleep one night, however much energy we invest. You will probably find yourself sobbing, crying, moaning, laughing, feeling lonely, distraught, abandoned and much more at some time on your voyage. All of these experiences and emotions have their place but they cost. For the individual who has spent a whole lifetime avoiding such emotional costs this can feel like a heavy price indeed.

Perhaps the biggest cost of all, however, is that which comes from overcoming our fears of intimacy. It is a paradox that most people actually fear the very things they most need in life, and this applies more to intimacy than to most. Our craving for intimacy in adult life often arises from our poor experiences with it in early life (see page 20). As adults we can therefore be terrified of trying yet again at something that we have, according to our unconscious, so badly failed at in the past. So it is that many of us actually sabotage our efforts and those of our partner while all the time asserting that what we really need is to experience more intimacy.

Creating intimacy has to be worked at, as we have seen. While we are making this effort, the possibility of success is ever present and can be very threatening. It is impossible to change a relationship without altering our life-style and some of these changes will be major ones if we are starting an intimate relationship from scratch. Most of us fear change, if only because, by definition, we cannot predict where it will lead us. Change in this area of life, however, is even more threatening because it takes us not only into new territory in the here-and-now but also into old experiences. Our old unconscious hopes and yearnings, so long held in check with varying degrees of success, now resurface along with the old pains of failure, or success, from our childhood. Dealing with this is not easy and has a price-tag.

Deeply embedded in all of this is the fear of loss. If we have nothing we cannot lose anything. Once we have something of great value, however, the more anxious we become that it might be taken away from us. The more intimate we become with our partner the more vulnerable we feel. At one level this is good because only by being this open can we be truly ourselves. Yet on the reverse of the coin is the danger of such vulnerability, which tells us that the more we open up the more we have to lose and the greater the likelihood is that we will be rejected once our real self becomes apparent. 'If you know me less you might love me more' is the sort of thing that goes through many people's minds at this time. 'If you really knew me, then you would know all the horrid parts of me; how insecure I am; how suicidal I feel sometimes; and then how *could* you love me?'

At this stage, many of us 'test the system'. We say to ourselves, usually quite unconsciously, 'Before I actually get too deeply into this intimacy business and lay myself open to you rejecting me once you see the real me, I will just test you a bit. I will begin with a simple test and, if you pass that, I will keep on making each test more difficult until you fail or leave.   Then I will have proved that I was right. You obviously do have limits to what is acceptable in me and now I have found them.' Such individuals can now console themselves with the fact that they were right all along and definitely should not put themselves at the risk of being abandoned.

The trouble is that, given human creativity and obstinacy, if we keep on testing anything to destruction we can usually achieve it. One-to-one relationships are no exception. All of this is, however, just an easy way out. We are acting out our fear of becoming intimate and so losing something that is dear to us. This is a self-ful-filling prophesy, however, because we can easily make ourselves so unlovable that our partner *will* reject us. What have we proved except that our old unconscious message on the subject was right? We have not grown; we have stayed immobile and frightened just as we were all those years ago in the cradle or whenever. No healing has taken place and we are destined to be lonely and in pain for ever.

We looked at commitment more on page 42, but here suffice it to say that a commitment to our partner or to our relationship in this context is really a com-mitment to ourselves. If we fail to make such a commitment we in fact abandon ourselves in a far more harmful way than our partner ever could. This sort of abandonment is a type of living death. The major characteristics of living things are that they change and grow. This is just as true of a blade of grass as it is of a complex human being. There is nothing wrong with death; all life is a preparation for it. What is unbearable for most of us, however, is living our death when we should be living our life.

There are, then, considerable costs involved in becoming more intimate. The dividend is usually well worth the investment, though, and for many individuals it is the most significant investment they will ever make in themselves. Such a human being now becomes a rich source of life for others around him or her and relationships at home, work and play take on a new lease of life. What at first appeared too costly now looks like a bargain. At the partnership level we invest one and our lover invests another one, but what we get out is usually at least three. The energy that can be created within a loving relationship can then multiply that three manifold and in ways that neither could have foreseen. This is the rich harvest that intimacy creates in the lives of those who are brave enough to pay the price of the entry ticket.

THE CHALLENGE OF CHANGE

Change, as we have seen, is unavoidable if we want to build a more intimate life. As most of us know, it is easy to see how others, especially our partner, should change. It is far more difficult to look into ourselves and address what needs changing there. In a sense this is what this book is all about.

We live in a fast-changing society that forces us to alter our attitudes and behaviour if we are to survive with any success. But one thing never changes: our fear of change itself. Most of us feel happiest with situations we know. Familiarity prevents us from having to redefine life on a day-by-day basis. After all, we have to be able to take certain things for granted or life would become intolerably unpredictable. It is probably true to say that today's society calls for too much change too quickly, and that many people are not well-equipped to deal with it.

Against this background many people feel they should at least be able to rely on their one-to-one relationship to be a steadying rock in their lives, something that will help them cope with the change all around them. How difficult it is, therefore, when such people discover that the rock they thought they could cling to turns out to be changing just as quickly and unpredictably as many other areas of their life. Set against this enormous rate of change and our fear of it, however, is an almost hypnotic desire to make changes. It is this balance of the desire to change and to stay as we are that creates so much friction in relationships between intimates.

When working with couples I often find that the whole subject of change gets off to a bad start because many believe they 'know' how their partner should change and are often equally certain about how they themselves should change. When we examine the issues more carefully, however, it turns out that the things that one or other partner thinks should be changed are the best parts of their personalities – the very traits that brought them together in the first place. This sort of problem comes about because most of us see our personality characteristics as being 'all good' or 'all bad'. Of course they are not. Even a partner's meanness, for example, can be turned to good advantage as he or she takes care of the finances.

Do not forget that we unconsciously choose one another on the basis of our differences. So it is that our very best traits can also be our worst and vice versa.

Do be cautious then when working through this book with your partner. Remember that few of us are all one thing or another and that our most annoying traits can often turn out to be the most rewarding in our relationship if we are conscious of what is going on and know how to harness them. In a loving and intimate relationship even very negative behaviour can sometimes be used to good advantage by the couple as they examine their attitudes to the greys of life rather than polarize everything into blacks and whites.

One of the biggest problems I come across in this area is that people can often see what change could or should be made but are terrified of starting on it because the task seems too big. I begin by encouraging such a couple to break down the apparently insurmountable hurdle into smaller units, each one of which can be tackled with ease. This creates confidence and makes everyone, myself included, optimistic and matters progress well. Such change, built as it is on small units of improvement, also tends to last longer than grand gestures that are made quickly but then collapse equally fast. Agreeing on what can be done and then achieving it with small building blocks almost always works best.

Many of us find we are stuck in our relationships, stuck, that is, in terms of growth and change. Some people tell me that this feels familiar to them and that their father, or whoever, was much the same for all his life. I tend to take a rather more challenging view on this by pointing out that change is one of the features of life itself. Even inanimate objects are in a process of change. So personal and interpersonal change is inevitable. It is only a matter of how we manage it. Many people see all change as largely threatening but a few regard it as a challenge. Those who are too close or too distant in their relationships cannot usually see the potential benefits of change and many couples fear that trying to change matters will make them less rather than more intimate.

As with so many areas of the emotional life, the paradoxes in all of this are huge. The openness and trust required of us if we are to change and grow as individuals or as a couple are the very meat and drink of true intimacy. One of the greatest barriers to increased intimacy is the inability or unwillingness to change. It might not be anything within the relationship itself that most needs changing. It might be our job; something long ago from our first family; something we need to forgive or be forgiven for; something we need to know more about so that we can understand it better; and so on. When trying to create and maintain a life together, we do not do this in isolation; it all takes place against the background of the rest of our lives as workers, parents, friends, family members and so on. Change in one of these areas can often help us be more intimate with our beloved.

So how you use what you have read in this part of the book will be largely up to you. Either you could choose to see it all as somewhat threatening, a task too great to embark upon or even something that you could not manage at all, or you could join in a journey of discovery with your partner, using one another as a vehicle for your own personal change. In doing this the relationship itself will change in a profound way that will, inevitably, lead to greater intimacy, both in and out of bed.

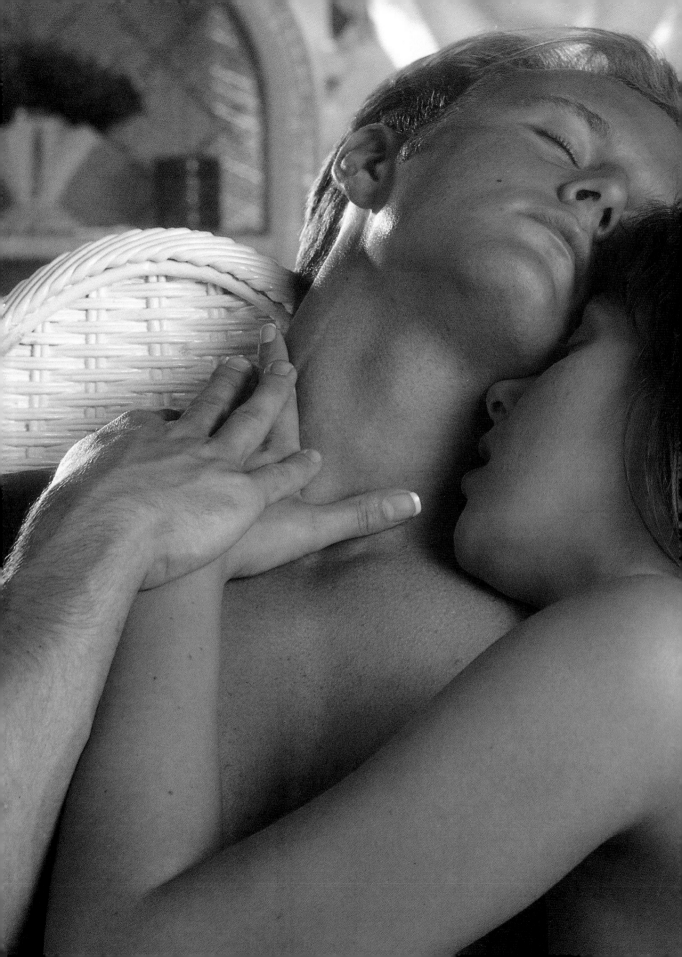

SEX AND INTIMACY

The link between sex and intimacy is a complex one. Many people immediately equate sex with intimacy but, as we have seen throughout the book so far, this is not helpful. It is possible to have quite good or even very rewarding sex with someone with whom we are not intimate, yet most people agree that sexual intercourse within an intimate relationship is often more meaningful. In this section we look at the direct links between sex and intimacy as a prelude to seeing how to make it all happen in Part Three.

We have considered the many faces of intimacy in Part One; now let us look at how all this interfaces with sex itself. Sex involves the merging of emotional and spiritual intimacies with physical ones. This brings pleasure and pain.

There are many 'dangers' in being intimate with anyone but once we introduce physical expressions of intimacy through sex into our relationship things become even more complex. Most of us fear hurt and rejection; a loss of individuality; that we might be taken over; that our faults might be exposed; that our lover might use private information to our disadvantage; and loss of control. Any or all of these can become barriers to intimacy between a couple outside the bedroom. They come into even finer focus once sex itself is involved.

It might be useful, first of all, to separate out the three main types of sexual experience between adults. The first is that sort of 'sex' that takes place between a couple, lovers or not, who are attracted to one another, even if they are not doing anything genital about it. In a sense this is a sort of prolonged foreplay – an overture to the first act of genital activity together – if one is to occur at all. This part of an existing couple's sexual life is highly personalized to them; reflects their relationship generally; may or may not be intimate at an emotional or spiritual level; and colours the sort of sex they have in bed. The notion I am trying to convey here is that a lot of 'sex' goes on between men and women, with or without intimacy, even if they are not currently, and may never be, lovers. Indeed some people are more capable of being intimate in such a setting than they are in a committed relationship that involves genital expressions of sex. Many work-place romances, opposite-sex friendships and dealings with others who are genitally unavailable are conducted in this style. In this way members of the opposite sex can be attracted to one another and be highly intimate yet not actually have sex. Some couples even run their marriages like this. This sort of 'non-genital' sex is still nonetheless serious sexual behaviour between two such individuals, as many of those who have had a non-sexual-intercourse affair can confirm.

The second type of sex is copulation. In this we get together to do actual genital business. Such a coupling, however, is possible with anyone; is largely self-centred; is solely a genital activity; is seen as an end in itself; requires only limited cooperation from our partner (his or her satisfaction is incidental to the whole exercise); tends to be stereotyped; has limited horizons; does not cope well with failure; calls for little or no revelation of one's self; and is content with short-term gains. Almost all sexual relationships start here and many continue in this way for a whole lifetime. Even very loving and intimate couples can enjoy sex at this level, if only from time to time. As we shall soon see, it is probably fair to say that more men than women enjoy sex of this kind though this is a huge generalization.

The third type of sex we can have is real intercourse. This is rather different

---

The couple who remain creative, experimental and open to change are most likely to experience true intercourse, as opposed to 'having sex'. Only real intimates can have intercourse, even if from time to time they have 'quickie' sex as a lusty change.

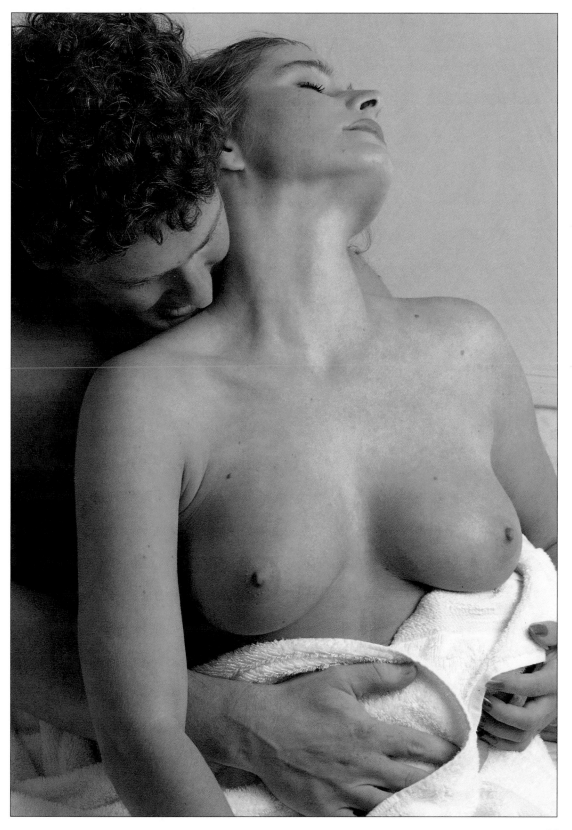

from copulation and is usually part of an intimate relationship, even if that relationship is brief. It could be argued that it is possible to have the sort of sexual intercourse I am describing in a very short-lived affair if one or both parties involved is already capable of intimacy. Sexual intercourse, as I see it, is personalized to our partner; is centred on the other person and his or her needs; is largely about interpersonal communication; is part of a couple's life-style together; takes our partner's needs into account; calls for considerable insight and imagination; enhances the value of our partner to us; can be varied according to the situation; has limitless horizons; copes well with failure; includes heart and soul as well as body; involves considerable self-revelation; assumes a knowledge of one another's secrets; tends to improve with time; and is a lifetime's investment.

We clearly stand a better chance of experiencing this sort of love-making in the context of an intimate relationship. It is important to bear in mind, however, that there is room for all three types of sex within a loving and intimate bond. Where problems occur, and what brings couples to me as a therapist, is that they can only ever experience one of the first two types. Understandably this feels somewhat superficial and leaves both partners dissatisfied at a deep level that, until the matter of intimacy is raised, cannot be named or identified. I believe that it is loveless, non-intimate copulation, for example, that makes so many men claim that they want more sex. When copulating they are spectating at their own 'love-making' and never really experience the transcendental joys of true sexual intercourse because they cannot let go. The search for a higher level of intimacy in the presence of another takes them on tedious and fruitless journeys around and around the sexual arena.

Many of the troubles that plague sexual intimacy start early in life in the way we raise girls and boys so differently when it comes to sex. We have looked at some of this already but here it might be useful to consider certain cultural stereotypes that hinder our journey towards more intimate sexual intercourse.

It has traditionally been claimed that women need to be in love or at least to feel something emotionally for their partner in order to have enjoyable sex. Such an assertion has brought with it a whole range of problems over the centuries. In recent decades, however, this has been turned on its head as females of all ages see their sexuality as being a much more free-standing commodity rather than something that a man (whom they love) 'does' to them. In my work as a therapist I find the distinction between 'women who will only have sex within an emotional setting' and 'men who can have sex with any female at any time' largely untrue and greatly damaging. Certainly many more women than men *say* that they want an emotional component to their sexual lives than do men but it would be foolish to be seduced into believing that this means that men want only a 'loveless fuck'. In fact nothing could be further from the truth, as we have seen in the section on men and intimacy (see page 67).

The problem is that boys are raised to see sex as a largely goal-centred 'performance' at which they have to 'succeed', as in so many other areas of life. The anxiety and tension that this creates, along with the very real expectation to obtain and maintain an erection if anything penetrative is to occur, often rules out emotional matters, or at best makes them more difficult. This is, to some extent, a biological difference between the sexes that is difficult to ignore. A woman can have enjoyable sex, and perhaps even an orgasm, if she simply lies there with her legs apart, being 'done to'. The male's role has to be more active, though, because without an erect penis nothing can happen. Whatever is said about loving foreplay, most people still see 'real sex' as involving penis-in-vagina activity.

This implicit and explicit performance concern makes any sort of sexual encounter more fraught, or at least potentially so, for men than for their partners. This then, coupled with the way boys and young men are reared to play down or deny their feelings, makes sex a more physical matter for men than it is for women. In a parallel way, being pregnant and having a baby is a more physically compelling activity for a woman than for her partner.

Raised as they have been in recent centuries, many women still put great emphasis on emotional connection during sex whereas men tend not to do so. When people ask me about this, and it is one of the commonest questions with which I am faced, I usually say something about sperms being cheap and eggs expensive and my questioner knows exactly what I mean. As cultural attitudes to sex change, however, there is more to this than the simple biological fact that females have babies and are therefore more likely to be interested in nurturing a relationship with any potential father of their children.

Today's woman is much more goal-centred in her sexual expression; can separate love and sex in a way that her grandmother could not have done; does not see her eggs as all that expensive because she can largely prevent unwanted pregnancy or abort a foetus she does not want; and so on. In fact most men today tell me that their women, and indeed females in general, seem to have considerable advantages when it comes to sex. Once we separate sexual intercourse from procreation and make it into a kind of recreational relationship builder, the balance of emotion and performance alters hugely. A woman in this model no longer sees herself as 'put upon' by a man who might or might not make sex enjoyable for her; and her man does not see himself as having to make all the running. The sexual relationships of the 1990s and beyond will be more evenly balanced with both partners taking responsibility for their own sexual expression and satisfaction.

These are major changes over a very short space of time and millions of couples are having problems coming to terms with them. Having said this, however, my experience is that most couples under the age of about forty are demolishing old barriers in a way that opens up their whole lives to greater intimacy than their parents, let alone their grandparents, would have thought possible. Many older people lament the fact that in earlier life they never really communicated with their partner, never said what they liked or wanted in bed, or indeed out of it, and so on. Many older people today, taking a lead from the young, enjoy an emotional and sexual life that is hugely better than they ever had in their previous thirty or forty years together. This is heartening at a time when we are living longer and as those in their sixties and beyond expect to remain sexually active if they have a partner. This blurring of boundaries between the sexual stereotypes of the past provides us with a fertile seed-bed for greater intimacy and hope for the next generation.

Continued on page 104

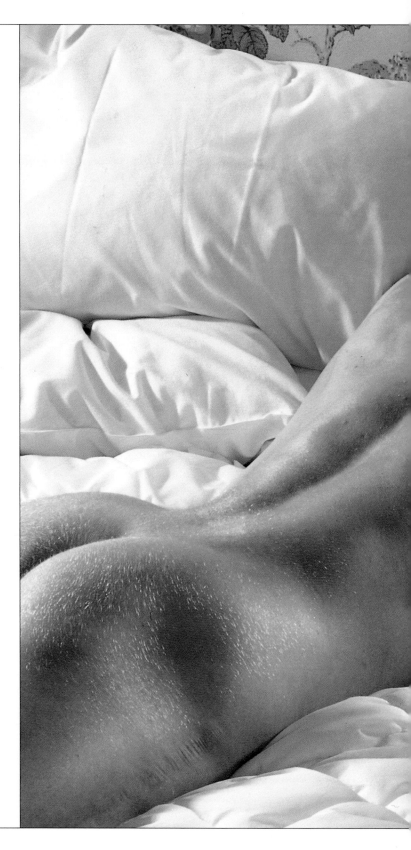

This woman clearly knows what she wants and is guiding her man to give it to her. Today's sexual relationships are much more equal when it comes to responsibility between the sexes. Younger women in particular ask for what they want and men are able to be more honest about their feelings. This balancing of responsibility in bed greatly helps a couple to be intimate as they cast off traditional sexual stereotypes in favour of being 'real'.

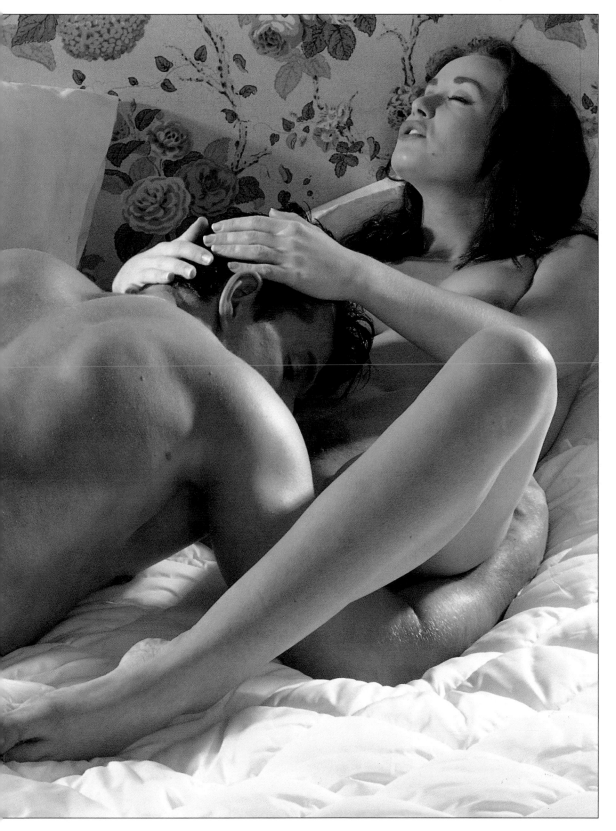

In describing the kind of intimate sexual life to which we could all aspire, I am not suggesting that this depth and intensity of experience is a constant or even consistent feature of the intimate relationship. The path of the sexually intimate relationship is littered with day-to-day events that make sexual intimacy difficult or even impossible to achieve. Couples who are really acquainted with intimacy and have an infrastructure of intimate behaviour within their relationship, however, can withstand even quite severe setbacks and still enjoy good sex. Such a relationship acknowledges and makes the best of angry sex, depressed sex, sad sex, lonely sex, and so on. These couples know that sex cannot always involve a touching of joyous souls. Indeed some of the most meaningful sexual experiences of intimate couples arise out of very unsexy experiences in daily life.

The beauty of an intimate relationship is that sex is allowed to emerge from all kinds of undercurrents both within the relationship and outside it. Against such a background there are no 'ideal' conditions in which 'perfect sex' occurs. Truly intimate couples can use their sexuality to express almost any emotion that they find themselves experiencing either alone or as a couple.

WHICH IS MORE IMPORTANT, SEX OR INTIMACY?

When women are asked which they would rather have, a superb sex life or a more intimate life generally, including physical intimacies short of intercourse, the majority choose the latter. Even some of my most recent studies, at a time when women are said to be more interested in sex than ever, have found that 'a good cuddle' is rated very highly by women, often in preference to intercourse itself.

Several studies show that most people, men and women, do not necessarily equate sexual satisfaction with marital satisfaction. One or two studies in fact have found that those who have the 'best marriages', as defined by the couple themselves, often have most 'sex problems'. On the other side of the coin are those who claim to have a terrible marriage but a very good sex life.

The link, therefore, between 'great sex' and happy, intimate relationships is far from simple. Clearly many couples of all ages have very intimate lives with little or no sex. In my work there is no direct link between how much a couple's sex life improves in therapy and how they view their partnership overall. Some people are delighted with increased intimacy whether or not it brings better sex and others find that improved sex enhances their whole intimate life together. It is almost impossible to give simplistic assurance to a couple starting therapy.

In general it is fair to say that women report less sexual satisfaction in their relationships than their men do. Also, husbands' and wives' definitions of sexual intimacy vary quite a lot, especially in older groups. Men in general find it easier to see their sex life as a separate entity within their partnership whereas their wife's

---

Learning to be intimate with oneself is the starting point to greater sexual intimacy with our lover. Many men see their body as unlovable and as a result cherish and value it little, if at all. More positive attitudes bear fruit in bedroom dealings with their lover.

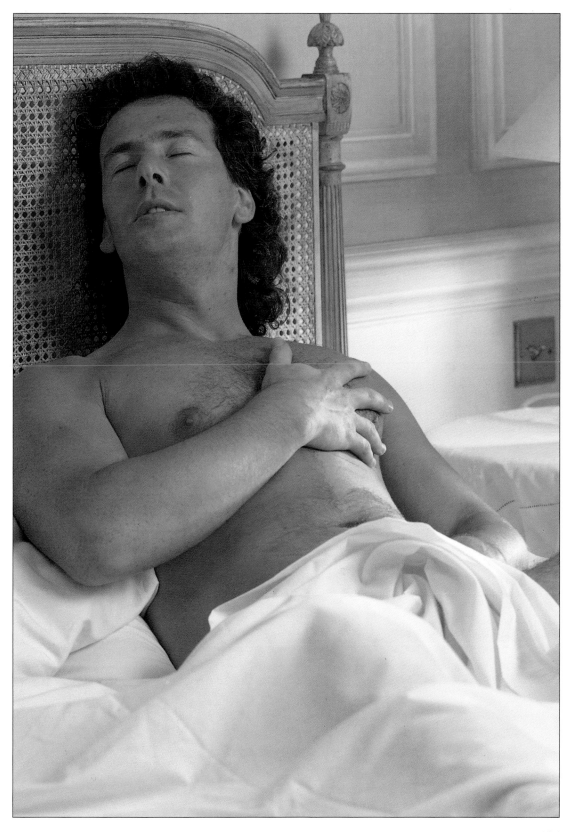

perception of her sexual life is usually more closely linked to the degree of intimacy within the whole relationship. By and large I find that if I want to get a true picture of the emotional state of any relationship it is better to ask the woman. Most men, for reasons that we looked at briefly on page 76, tend to play down any issue that might threaten their love bond because it is so much more valuable to them than to their partner. Men also tend to focus more widely on other issues in life and put their emotional relationship relatively low on their agenda – at the conscious level – at least until it is threatened. Then they are just as keen to see it survive, perhaps even more so, than their wife is. On a day-to-day basis, though, most men take their relationship for granted provided that they are getting the sex, nurturing and servicing they want.

Which partner's perception of the relationship is the more accurate is open to debate. It could be that we have traditionally raised girls in our culture to have unrealistic expectations and thus to be too emotionally demanding of their one-to-one partnership. This, rather than men being hopeless as intimates, could be at the heart of so many women's dissatisfaction with their intimate life, and thus their sex life. Perhaps men's ability to separate sex from the whole relationship has its advantages as well as its drawbacks. Indeed this model is being adopted by increasing numbers of women, especially younger ones. Another advantage is that sex seen as more of a stand-alone product is not as vulnerable to the daily fluctuations in intimacy that are inevitable in modern life. If, on the other hand, it becomes a substitute for intimacy, it can easily degenerate into loveless copulation. This benefits neither partner.

Perhaps, as with so many of these issues, we should take a broad view and look at the sum total of pleasure and reward within any individual relationship. For the woman it might be that she largely enjoys the emotionally intimate elements whilst putting a relatively low priority on the genital ones; for her man the opposite might apply. Taken as a whole, though, both could enjoy a tolerable balance, which ends up at approximately the same satisfaction 'score', albeit via different routes. After all, whoever said that men and women should be the same?

Sex is highly emphasized in current Western culture. It is unashamedly sold to the young and expectations run high from before the first time we have sexual intercourse. The level of intimacy experienced during the sex act itself can be so high that it lures women especially into believing that it could be available for much more of the time they spend with their man. This is probably unrealistic.

The trouble with any discussion of all this is that there is considerable variation between couples and even within the same couple as the years pass. I often address these issues with very different couples, even in the same working day. In one session, for example, I could be dealing with a young couple who both see sex as paramount. The woman might be highly assertive, going for what she wants, and appearing to behave more like a male in her attitudes to sex and intimacy. In the next session with another couple, perhaps in their fifties, the wife comes out with all the stereotypical complaints about him 'always wanting sex' whilst her husband maintains that she is interested only in 'cuddling and being emotional'. What is certain, though, is that few couples break up solely because of a dissatisfaction with their sexual life. Nearly three-quarters of all divorces in the Western world are initiated by women and the most common complaint has to do with problems with communication and other intimacy issues. Studies show that couples who can communicate both verbally and emotionally cope well with even very poor levels of *sexual* intimacy. It is important to remember too that many couples stay together for reasons that have nothing to do with intimacy *or* sexual satisfaction and that for some a poor relationship is better than no relationship at all.

Perhaps an issue worth looking at here is that of 'free sex'. Many of us imagine that once we get married, or start to live with someone, sex will be 'free'. Alas this is not so. Sex, in a sense, is never free – it always costs. Some of the highest prices are venereal diseases, including the potentially fatal AIDS; and unwanted pregnancy. Down the list come items such as financial cost, emotional and relationship costs, and so on. Many uncommitted sexual dalliances leave people with a sense of loss, guilt, shame, fear, or shabbiness. Sex can also easily seduce us into a relationship that creates expectations of the future that are totally unrealistic and harmful to us. Here the price that we pay for the sex we enjoy can be horrendous. Except within a very intimate relationship, there is no such thing as sex without a price, however subtle the price and no matter when we are called upon to pay.

For young people, sex can force them to engage in intimate relationships for which they are not ready and which can actually harm them. The intimate life is one that we should freely and intelligently choose, not something that we should rush into on the roller-coaster of sexual thrills. Many a young, head-over-heels couple will spend more time in one another's company in a day than the average happily married couple would spend in a week or more. Often the relationship cannot stand the strain. But no one ever warns the young about this cost.

Those who find themselves overtaken by genital intimacies usually say with hindsight that they grew very little at the time and were actually inhibited from being intimate. The trouble is that, however good sex is, we simply cannot spend twenty-four hours a day doing it. Even with the most creative minds at work, genitally expressed sexual intimacies can only take us so far. Recent decades of sex manuals suggest that sex is the best way to obtain more intimacy but millions of people have discovered that this is a false promise. Certainly it can increase our value to one another in bed and even, to some extent, out of it, but too much time and energy spent focusing on sexual intercourse means there is less to invest elsewhere in our relationship. This unwitting flight from intimacy suits many of those whose previous experiences of intimate relationships have been disappointing or worse. So it is that those of us who were most damaged in our formative years find ourselves grasping for more and better sex in the hope that we will find the intimacy we crave. It is a fruitless search.

Quality, in a sense, is more important than quantity when it comes to sex and quality comes from time and effort spent learning about one another and oneself. Sex against this sort of background costs relatively little because it is born out of real intimacy. All other efforts at 'better sex' are usually rooted in unconscious (or sometimes conscious) manipulation and control of our partner. By making him or her feel guilty, using threats, inducing fears, punishing, and in many other ways,

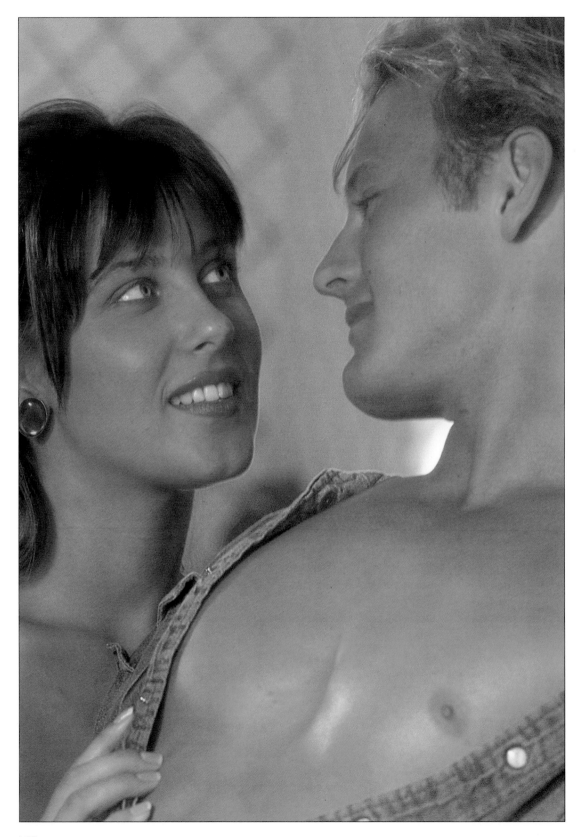

we try to force our lover to do or be what we want. The cost to the relationship is obviously very high. Women have in the past been trained to use sex as a weapon at worst or a bargaining chip at best. In a monogamous relationship a woman can indeed wield considerable power by withholding sex or love or by handing it out as a reward if her partner has behaved as she wishes. To use sex in these ways is clearly destructive to any relationship, yet even today some mothers tell their girls, directly or indirectly, to behave in this way. As men see their worth as closely linked to their sexual performance and express their intimate and loving life genitally, they cannot stand much of this sort of bribery, bullying and bartering. They become very angry. Such anger is acted out, usually unconsciously, in many ways outside the bedroom, by controlling the finances, for example. Although money is less of an issue these days than it was in the past, most couples still have profound disagreements over how it should be spent, and sometimes even over how it should be earned. Men, used to having quite a lot of power in this area of life, now find that they have less, and this, coupled with women's increased sexual demands makes many feel disempowered in their relationships. After all, money and sex were the two major arenas in which, until recently, they had wielded most of their power. Many of the sexually dysfunctional men I see are consciously or unconsciously acting all this out, making their partner pay a sexual or emotional price for her behaviour. After all, no one can argue with a limp penis, so such a man has the ultimate trump card. A couple playing games such as these are clearly not being as intimate as they could. With care and skill, however, they can change their expensive love-making into something much less costly.

It might be valuable to sit down one day and think what you *charge* for sex in your relationship. Do this on your own first and then share your ideas with your partner if you think you can. Does your model virtually assure failure? Are you driven by stereotypical ideals? Next, ask yourself what sex *costs* you personally. Do you feel guilty, inadequate, put down, labelled, dissatisfied, tired and under continual sexual demands? If so, sex could be costing you too much and you are probably already finding your own unconscious ways of avoiding it. Seek professional help with this if any of it is too deeply rooted to be dealt with by the two of you. This may well be the case if things have been going wrong for some time.

It can also be helpful to look at what sex means in your relationship. Talk about how important, or not, sex is to you as a way of expressing intimacy. When did you last talk about your sexual preferences and how they differ from those of your partner? I know this is difficult to do, especially in a committed, one-to-one relationship, but it is well worth doing. Try to find the common ground you share and build on it. You will find that working through the exercises in Part Three of this book will also help.

Building a quality of life that includes intimacy means spending time
together learning about our lover and ourselves. The more important task,
as we have seen, is learning about ourselves. Our lover is, or should be,
our best ally in this journey of self-discovery.

TURNING THE CLOCK BACK

Once we start to look at the physical intimacies of sex, as opposed to the emotional and spiritual ones, we cannot go far without discovering the intensely regressive nature of sexual intercourse. Our erotic and sexual lives begin in the womb. There is little doubt that spontaneous erections occur in unborn baby boys and baby girls must have similar experiences. Every mother of a male child will have seen her little son's penis erect when it is washed, touched or stimulated in some other way. Almost all of us who are parents have seen a child masturbate, albeit often indirectly by rocking, or in other ways stimulating their genitals whilst going red in the face and perhaps puffing and panting a little. Clearly, then, babies and young children experience countless erotic sensations, some of which involve their genitals.

We saw on page 28 that mothers interact differently with boys and girls right from birth. Many women are fascinated by the little penis and body of their 'man-child'. Girls are not the subject of such erotic fascination. This produces the results we saw on page 24. The vast majority of the attention we receive in early babyhood is, however, not genital at all. It involves caressing, cuddling, feeling safe, feeling loved, breast play, bathing with our parents, being dressed and undressed, and so on. All of these can be, and often are, experienced as 'erotic' in the widest sense of the word yet they are not directly genital. As we get older we take over a lot of these basic caring and nurturing activities from our parents and learn to do them for ourselves. The next time we consciously visit the erotic pleasures of these activities, most of which lie in our unconscious, is when we start to date. We now re-experience the pleasures and delights of being 'mothered' and nurtured. But now there is the added thrill of the very obvious genitally erotic effect that such physical intimacies produce. Old, largely unconscious memories of similar erotic joys from the past emerge and we relive the reality of them, for good or bad, with our girlfriends or boyfriends.

As we introduce sex into our petting, genitally orientated connections with the past become increasingly apparent. It seems ridiculous to me, working as I do with regression techniques, to assert that erotic pleasures and pursuits originate after puberty when our sex hormones take a hold of us. True, most of us enter a whole new world of sexual expression after puberty, but most of the territory has already been mapped in early life.

A mature sexual relationship, then, is mainly a replay and embellishment of the erotic experiences we have collected over a whole lifetime, from the cradle to the present day. This is important when thinking about physical intimacy because the individual who has a data bank of good experiences behaves differently from one who has not. When we make love we re-enact the separation-unity conflict that dogged us as a baby and young child. The actual physical activities also have

Much of adult love-making is a re-enhancement of unconscious pleasures from the past. This man is reliving the pleasures of his mother's breast and his partner is, in turn, rehearsing how to use her breasts to pleasure her own babies. And so the cycle continues.

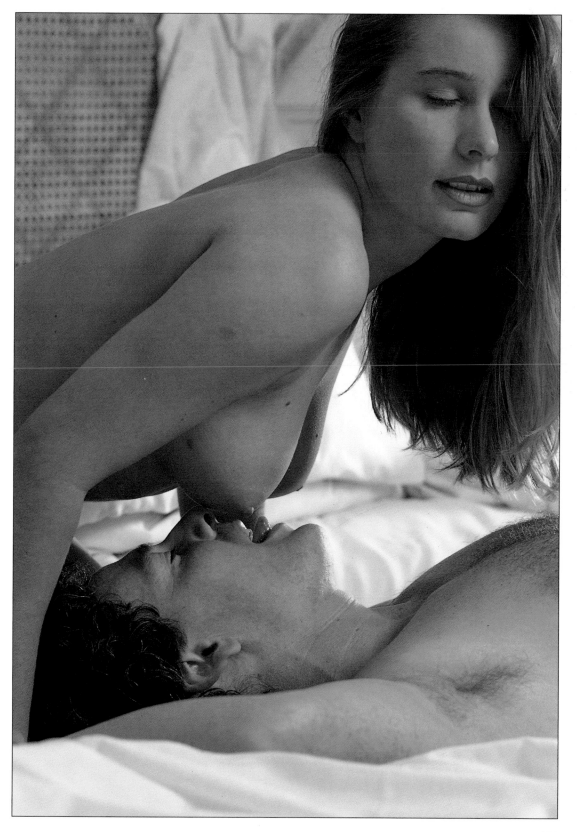

considerable significance. First, a man enters a woman. In a sense this takes him back to the womb – the last time that he was 'inside' a woman. It has been suggested that a man's deep thrusting and high levels of pleasure as he forces himself into his lover are a kind of primitive effort to regain entry to the womb, however symbolically. Certainly there is no other situation in life in which human beings 'get inside' each other, as babies are in the womb.

This joy of returning to the wet, warm environment of the loved female is, however, tainted by a fear of becoming a part of someone again, of being engulfed, of losing selfhood and hard-won individuality, as defined by society. So sex is, at this unconscious level, tinged with negative emotions for a man, especially if his previous experiences were of being overwhelmed by his mother as a baby. For the man whose memories are positive, this return to the 'safe womb' of his special woman can be the most intimate engagement he will ever know as an adult. Perhaps it is for this reason that so many men yearn for sex when in fact what they are really seeking is the re-enactment of this primal oneness. This love-hate relationship with sex draws men into it time and again in the unconscious hope of getting in touch with the feeling that they find so difficult even to come close to in any other sphere of life.

Women have things somewhat easier in a way because they are enabled by their biology and by society to touch with this sort of intimacy during their experiences of pregnancy, giving birth, child care and breast-feeding. They also have permission in our culture to do very intimate emotional business with other women. Men, in contrast, are somewhat impoverished.

For the average woman, then, the act of taking a man into her body, though hugely intimate at one level, is not quite as significant as the reciprocal process for a man. Many women have told me that the best thing about sex at a physical level is the sensation of 'being filled up'. Perhaps, given the desire to get away from their mother in a symbolic sense (see page 24), women would not want to 'get back into the womb' in their sexual dealings with a man, even if men had wombs. Rather they are more interested in expressing their most primal forms of physical intimacy by using their vagina to incorporate their partner. Perhaps this stems from an unconscious desire to love, nurture or mother him in the closest way that they can other than by actually having him inside their womb. Having dealt with many women over the years who have problems using their vagina positively during intercourse, and listening to the effects that this has on them at a very primitive level, I cannot believe for a moment that sex for a woman is simply about taking a man's penis into her vagina.

Whether or not female fans of oral and anal sex have a greater than average desire to incorporate their partner into their body is open to debate but I have considerable experience of these issues from working through them with my female patients. One woman recently told me, for example, that she felt she had at last lost her virginity in a profoundly meaningful way after having anal sex for the first time. For her, and for many like her, vaginal intercourse is certainly intimate, but in anal and oral sex such women touch within themselves a level of erotic completeness that is not possible through vaginal containment alone. Closely linked to all this is the powerful, negative message with which females particularly are burdened concerning anality. Countless women carry with them a 'tightness', both real and symbolic, in their pelvic and rectal muscles. This undoubtedly arises from over-strict potty-training in early life and the far greater emphasis put on females of all ages to 'be clean'. Many women confuse their rectum with their vagina in this respect and shut off their 'drain-like' vagina along with their tight anus. Boys, it appears, are not brought up to be nearly as concerned with cleanliness and, as a result, are less negative about their anal area and its erotic connections. If sex is 'dirty' to many women, how much more dirty is any erotic experience involving the anus or rectum, yet it is a biological fact that the anus is highly erotic in most people. It is hardly surprising then that so many women say that they are only prepared to indulge in oral or anal sex – both of which are more 'dirty' than ordinary sex – if they feel exceptionally 'intimate' with a man. To be fair, many men say exactly the same thing.

My experience of being with women while they are giving birth leaves me in no doubt that it is an intensely sexual process. Some women say that it is the biggest orgasm they have ever had and there are countless women who enjoy considerable stretching of their vagina during love-play, perhaps by their partner's fingers or whole hand. The very resistance that this remark produces in some women alerts me at once to the possibility that it is highly attractive yet unconsciously censored. By and large we train girls in our culture to get little pleasure from their vagina. A therapist such as myself sees countless women who get precious little joy at all from their genitals. Most have never been physically intimate with themselves and many have not incorporated their vagina into their body image. It is hardly surprising that such women find it difficult or impossible to be physically intimate with a man once they get beyond kissing and cuddling. Indeed, whilst it might seem somewhat provocative, I would assert that many women put the emphasis they do on *emotional* intimacy in their sexual life because they are at some level afraid to admit that they very much want overwhelming genital experiences, yet feel so ambivalent about them. Even women with quite good sex lives, as defined by them, often find that they get only a fraction of the pleasure and sense of transcendental connection of which they are capable. Once they jump the barriers created by their internal policeman and abandon themselves to 'being filled up', be it orally, anally or vaginally, their sexual life takes on a whole new quality.

Many of the problems that arise on such a journey towards ultimate sexual intimacy derive from the odd Western notion that sex is about a man penetrating a woman. Almost all sex is described as the man being the penetrator, the one who uses a 'weapon' (his penis) somehow to 'attack' or 'invade' his partner. The problems that arise from such a model are all too obvious.

I find it much healthier and more attractive to think of sexual intercourse as a highly intimate act in which a woman takes her man into her body. This now becomes a welcoming process of merging or engulfment rather than a threatening invasion. If it were possible to change society's use of language in this way then the sex act would also change, becoming a somewhat different type of pursuit. A woman would then be able to acknowledge that she enjoys sexual intercourse

113

because of what she gains by incorporating the body of another; and the man would not feel that he were somehow intruding on her person in what could be construed as a very non-intimate way. Language and attitudes are closely linked and as long as we describe sex in combative terms, men and women in general will never be able to be truly intimate in bed. Perhaps the highly intimate couple have, in their own way, overcome this cultural barrier so that she can symbolically incorporate him and he her, whether or not they are having sex.

It is perhaps interesting to mention here that there might be a biological 'need' or drive for females to contain things, albeit in a symbolic way for much of the time. In studies that looked at how pre-school children of both sexes created drawings, it was found that more girls than boys spontaneously enclosed their subjects within a border or outline. In the way that females of most ages form networks there is also a tendency to be inclusive, to involve others and to contain emotions within such groups. Linked to this are the deferred bodily pleasures of pregnancy and even childbearing. These are pursuits that call for long periods of 'being' rather than goal-centred 'doing'. Many women tell me, often in disguised ways of which they are unaware, that they defer pleasure quite regularly. Social examples abound that cannot, I believe, simply be explained by women's second-class position in society for so long. Perhaps this is one reason why female sexual arousal is a longer affair than that of the male. Could it be that most women 'contain' their arousal, keeping it to themselves as a personal experience, rather like having a baby in the womb, the more to relish it before 'giving birth' to their orgasm?

Whatever the explanation, and there is space to look at the subject only very simply here, I believe that women get maximum pleasure and fulfilment from all sorts of 'containment', be it emotional, spiritual or sexual. This might help explain why many women's biological and perfectly healthy desire to 'contain' gets so out of balance that they cannot let go at all. In a symbolic sense they are permanently pregnant but never give birth – permanently sowing but never reaping.

The physical side of sexual intimacy within any individual is clearly a complex collection of contradictory emotions, both conscious and unconscious. Whilst the encounter is somewhat different for the sexes, it is mostly complementary. This is why good sex is so powerful. We cannot hope to experience alone the joys to be had in the giving and taking involved. Sexual relief through masturbation, perfectly valid as a release in its own right, is a poor relative of intimate sexual intercourse involving, as it does, the touching of souls of those who know and love one another. Copulation, again perfectly acceptable as a stand-alone pastime, also falls short. The secret of a fulfilling sexual life is almost certainly the ability to balance these three types of sexual outlet, if one has a partner with whom to do so, so that we can be intimate with ourselves in masturbation; can experience the self-centred joy

---

Being open enough to masturbate in our partner's presence calls
for real trust. It is not just a matter of selfishly enjoying ourselves in his
or her presence: such openness enables soul-to-soul contact that is
invaluable for the whole relationship.

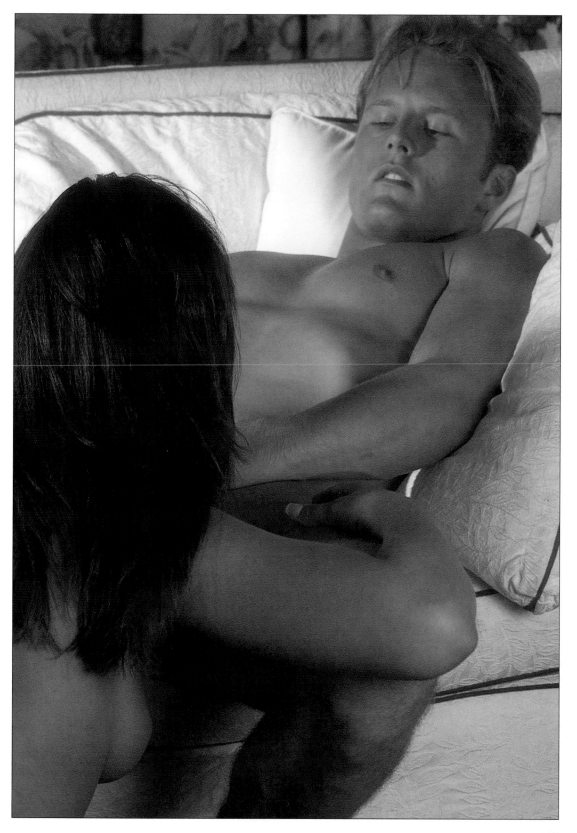

of copulatory relief with a partner; and can be sufficiently intimate to abandon ourselves to the total regressive, unnameable delights of sexual intercourse. In so doing we come to 'know' ourselves in the presence of our lover and to experience real intimacy.

When we 'make' love we are in a very real sense making something tangible. We are going back into our data bank of physically intimate experiences and reliving them step by step. In so doing we re-enact our courtship days; feel excited as if we were meeting our beloved for a teen date; discover the joys of masturbation in his or her presence; seek and hopefully find the peace and acceptance of babyhood as we make up sexy languages and baby-talk; touch and are touched; use our whole bodies, skin-to-skin, just as we did with our mother; suck at the breast; make baby-like noises; dress and undress one another with all its attendant arousal; and so on. These physical intimacies trigger the unconscious spiritual and emotional intimacies from the past that we unconsciously associate with them. This is what makes adult love-making so compelling, fulfilling and rewarding. There is no other arena in which, as adults, we can regress to those glorious days when we felt so deliciously erotic in the hands of someone who unconditionally loved us.

In this way physical intimacy in adult life catapults us into long-'forgotten' transcendental states of bliss. We lose contact in these moments with the real world with all its worries and burdens and abandon ourselves in trust to the flood of sexual experiences that are physical, emotional and spiritual.

To claim that females want or need this any more than males do is mistaken. The dilemma, if indeed there is one in any particular couple, is how to empower men so that they can relax enough from performance-centred issues in the bedroom and get the best out of physical intimacies. Perhaps then, having handed over some of the responsibility to his partner, such a man could free himself to engage with her emotionally in a way that is impossible or unlikely when he has the whole burden of sexual 'performance' on his shoulders. In this way the man who is constantly asking himself 'How am I *doing*?' might be able to consider 'How am I *being*?'.

Whether all this should start with greater intimacy at a non-genital level out of the bedroom is not a debate that I wish to join. Many women claim that they would be much better in bed if their man were more 'intimate', by their definition, out of it. On the other hand, many males say that they would feel freer to be significantly more intimate if they were playing on a level field, which they are not. Such men complain that their women want them to be great emotionally *and* wonderful physically yet that they, the women, do not pull their weight in bed when it comes to physical intimacies.

My experience with younger couples is that much of this debate is becoming sterile. Most young couples today take a more equal responsibility for their loving life both in and out of bed. Indeed, the sort of intimate life that you can build by following the precepts of this book has few boundaries between the bedroom and the outside world. Whilst many women say that foreplay should start the minute they get up if their man wants them to be receptive at ten o'clock that night, it should, in fairness, also be said that such women should be more physically and genitally contributory through the day if their man is to feel that they are reciprocating. Once this sort of balance is created or restored in a couple's life, then both contribute to the emotional *and* physical intimacies they want and do so in and out of the bedroom in a way that blurs the division between the two.

When I talk about all this with couples I describe a life-style that consists of 'making love all day'. At first they think I am crazy but soon come to understand that true sex, real intercourse, as opposed to copulation, is simply one part of a love-making pyramid. At the base are the hosts of little loving and caring activities, both physical and emotional, that make life pleasant. Here we hold hands in a shop, kiss for no reason, take care of one another emotionally and interact in the way that I have described in Part One. The next slice of the pyramid involves more physical intimacies such as cuddling, breast-play, massaging one another, deep kissing, and so on. Arousal may or may not be the aim but at this level we are more physically intimate than we would be with a good friend. The third level of physical intimacy involves genital arousal and, hopefully, emotional and spiritual connection, if the couple is intimate. At the very top of the pyramid is sexual intercourse itself. If you were to draw up such a diagram for yourself you would soon see that the biggest areas by far are those at the bottom of the structure. Sexual intercourse is only a tiny fraction of the area of the pyramid, occupying as it does, only the peak. It sits, however, on the other intimate experiences we enjoy and without them has no foundation. Most of the exercises in Part Three are really aimed at creating a better pyramid so that you have a good foundation on which to place your love-making pinnacle.

The couple with such a solid pyramid finds that journeys from one level to another are easy and free from friction and debate. Such couples find that a cuddle at the right moment and in the right setting can be just as 'intimate' as full-blown sex and that all the pieces that comprise the pyramid interlock to form their own unique jigsaw of intimacy. Where 'sex' starts and finishes in all this is somewhat academic: such couples are 'making love' all the time, whether it happens to involve their genitals or not.

This, it seems to me, is what intimacy is about at the sexual level. Much of what I described in Part One could be applied to any relationship at work, with friends, in the family or at play. The sexually intimate pyramid, though, is very different in that we choose to build it and live it with one special person. Sexual intercourse itself is also a unique human experience, unlike anything we do with even our closest friends, and this colours the whole nature of the pyramid.

So far so good. But we do not come to our one-to-one relationship with a clean slate. We have not all had loving and intimate childhoods. Most of us are at least somewhat 'wounded' or damaged by our upbringing and are seeking someone with whom we can remedy this. The minute we start to build our sexual pyramid, therefore, the workforce is hampered by old, largely unconscious, notions that may have lain dormant since babyhood. Now our neediness starts to intrude and to affect, possibly adversely, our efforts to create and maintain a sexually intimate life together. Old fears, guilt, shame, rages, anger, humiliations, punishments, and so on, rear their heads as we expect our lover to behave in the way our personal data bank tells us our intimate parent or carer did – or should have done. So it is that we half expect to be let down; to be abandoned; to be told off; to be found wanting; or to be too much or too little of something or other. Against this background the tiniest problem in the here-and-now can grow to become a real horror.

All of this is made more difficult because in our culture we try to remain faithful to one sexual partner at a time. If he or she appears to be activating painful circuits from the past, making us feel wretched, a sexual failure, or whatever, we are stuck in a way that we are not in other areas of life where other alternatives are open to us. Also, given that most of us have only a tiny number of sexual partners compared with the numbers of experiences we have in most other areas of life, we have little to compare with and so do not really know what *we* are contributing to the current problems and what is our partner's business. This not knowing what is 'normal' plagues many a couple's sex life and often leads them to look outside their one-to-one relationship for answers. Unfortunately, solutions are not easy to come across because 'normal' when applied to sex is a range and not a point. Also, unlike when buying a washing-machine, it is often impossible for us to separate out our own unconscious business from that of our partner except by working on it over some time. And, unlike the washing-machine, both we and our partner are changing all the time.

Most problems with sexual intimacy arise in our unconscious pasts and the very road that can lead us to rediscovering the joys of past erotic intimacies can also take us in to old pains. This is why sex is such a minefield and yet at the same time such an avenue for healing. Having said this, my clinical experience suggests that true healing occurs only within intimate sexual relationships, not within the 'loveless fuck'. We do not need to be having 'healing' sex all the time, either with all of our sexual partners over a lifetime or within a long-term relationship, but neither should we be harming ourselves or our partner by doing 'bad' sexual business. Many of us unwittingly do this time and again with various partners. In this sense, then, good sex is a fight that engages our old unconscious material as we try to work it through in the here-and-now with our beloved. All our previous intimate and sexual experiences from childhood and adult life are in the melting pot as we make love *now*. This is why I suggest that couples go back to the bottom of the pyramid if they want to start to build an intimate sexual life together. Bolting on new 'optional extras' to a dilapidated car does not make it go any better and certainly does not prolong its life.

An interesting example of this was a woman I saw recently. We started on the bottom slice of the pyramid and at once ran into trouble. She could not even hold her husband's hand in public. The open demonstration of her sexuality that this involved was far too intimidating. This led to considerable discussion of other areas of their life together as we started to discover her previously unexamined concerns about sex in general. This tiny social-intimacy problem led us into minefields that were able to be traversed after only a few weeks. To this woman, it transpired, sex was so 'private' that it was too private even for their marital bedroom!

Being aware of our past, then, helps us to understand better where we are coming from in our intimate dealings with one another. Such awareness also explains, in my clinical experience, all kinds of otherwise baffling behaviour, beliefs and dilemmas. As we are composed of all our yesterdays, a greater understanding of our own and our partner's past can only lead to a more rewarding present.

SEX AND LOVE

I am always wary of discussing the subject of love because it means such different things to different people. Even one individual's definition of love can change over the years and it is a brave person who would claim to distinguish between love and intimacy. Most of us could have lusty sex with almost anyone: the copulation I have already referred to. In a perverse way this sort of copulation can have an intimacy about it in that both people are being truly themselves. On the reverse side of the coin, many a bedroom crime has been committed in the name of 'true love'. Loveless and lusty sex can also be a good starting point for intimate sex. It would be an unwise couple who waited until their relationship was deeply intimate before having intercourse, or even sex, if only because either can help us on our journey to intimacy.

When we are making love we have two tasks, in a sense. The first is making love to ourself and the second is making love to and with our beloved. Sex that was entirely 'me' based would be masturbatory, yet sex focused solely on our lover would be entirely 'other' based, would lack passion and would certainly not involve looking after ourselves and looking after our lover. At orgasm, and in the immediate run-up to it, we become self-centred, concentrating solely on our own pleasure and arousal. That we are doing this in the physically intimate presence of our beloved makes it all the more special, particularly if he or she is doing the same. This makes sex an almost unique arena in which to experience the difference between closeness and intimacy. If you have had intimate sex during which you have been aware not only of yourself but also sensitive to your lover then you will feel lovingly close to him or her. In this way your intimacy is enhanced by your closeness. Sex falls short when we focus on the 'me' or 'I'. Being intimate in sex enables us to be more passionate, more truly ourselves with our beloved.

This balancing of closeness – being exquisitely aware of you – with intimacy – being truly aware of me – is the very heart of rewarding sex. I do not want to masturbate using your body but I do not want to focus only on you and your pleasure either. If I am passionate it does not mean that I am unaware of you but my passion communicates to you and frees you to be more you. This authentic experience of intimacy during sex is so powerful that even if it is experienced only every now and again it glues us together and enables us to put up with the gritty task of working out our differences. This touching of souls, however infrequent, cannot be *un*known once we have experienced it. It takes us beyond the instinctual sort of sex in which animals engage to a connection that transcends normal interpersonal dealings. This, I believe, fuels the boiler of life together in a way nothing else can.

Sex, with all its metaphors of death and rebirth, also gives us an opportunity to live through these deepest of human experiences in a safe haven. Many people, women especially, claim that having an orgasm is like a 'little death' and that after

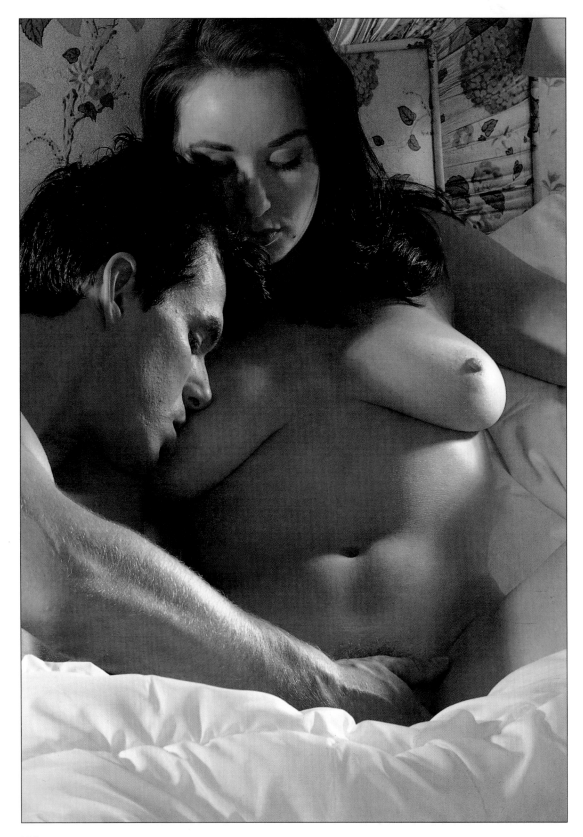

sex they feel reborn in some way. The loss of self-awareness, the other-worldliness of total arousal and the abandonment of our conscious selves is, in effect, a sort of death during sexual intercourse. It is probably the only situation in which we can experience an ending without a sense of loss or separation. This happens because very soon after the symbolic 'death' of orgasm we are resurrected to a new life with our beloved. Now we feel more loved, more connected, more alive, even though we have 'died'. In this way, I believe, we act out our real death but in sex we cheat it. It is also possible to say to one another, 'We did it together', and then to start afresh.

This mystical business that *is* sexual intercourse enables us to deal with the pains of pairing with our shadow. I cannot think of any other human activity that comes anywhere near achieving this. In connecting our death with our birth through condensing our intimate experiences of a lifetime into a few minutes, we dose ourselves with a drug that the pharmaceutical industry would give a king's ransom to own.

ALTERNATIVES TO PHYSICAL INTIMACY

For many people, the sort of love-making I have just described is, sadly, a fairy-tale dream. They have been so damaged by their personal childhood or later years, or by the culture in general that they cannot experience even quite simple physical intimacies, like the woman who could not hold her husband's hand in public. This level of guilt, fear and shame about sex that abounds in the unconscious of our culture is hard to over-estimate. This precludes millions of people from enjoying even quite simple kinds of intimacy because their 'internal policeman' never goes off duty. As human animals, however, we crave intimacy at the physical level and will seek it out in various symbolic ways if it is otherwise unavailable or if we cannot allow ourselves to have it directly. In this way millions of people misuse copulation, for example, as a substitute for sexual intercourse.

Some people find the physical intimacy they need in contact with professionals who offer it. Hairdressers, masseurs, doctors, fitness trainers, dance teachers and physiotherapists are just a few examples of professionals who dispense physical intimacy. Such relationships are usually 'clean' emotionally yet they still answer some of our physical needs. In fact the professional nature of such physical intimacies protects many people from going deeper. Although the threat of taking physical intimacy further is always there, strict boundaries are set both by the professionals and the consumers so that the latter can get what they need and want yet stay within acceptable boundaries. This has considerable value in a culture such as that in most Anglo-Saxon countries, where many people need much more physical intimacy than can be supplied by their partner – assuming they have one.

A balancing of closeness and intimacy is at the very heart of good
sex. This involves being sufficiently at ease with our body so that the
practicalities of sexual contact do not intrude adversely to prevent
the deep connectedness we seek.

As this sort of ritualized relationship with 'intimate professionals' carries with it at least some fear of sexual 'danger', however, we more often turn to other sources of physical contact to enhance our lives and make up for the deficits. In the UK and the USA there is a history of making domestic pets our most intimate non-human companions. Millions of people have pets in all Western societies. For some people, their relationship with their animal friends is more intimate than any with their human partners and acquaintances. There have been cases of women committing suicide after the death of a pet.

A pet provides something to care for, to cuddle and stroke, to treat like a baby and to kiss. Most of all, though, it loves us unconditionally: the very bedrock of all intimate relationships. Various studies have found that caressing a pet reduces blood pressure and/or heart rate but none has proven any sustained health benefits from pet ownership. What has been found, though, is that those who have a strong relationship with a pet cope with life's negative events better than those without one. A 1991 study found that positive changes in health occurred in people who acquired pets, though the researchers could not explain why this should be. Dog ownership appeared to be especially beneficial when compared with cat ownership but other studies have found that even pets such as fish can have positive effects.

Although most of us see our pets for the animals they are, some individuals see them as furry *people*. Indeed, in several societies pets are more pampered than are humans and it is fair to say that some individuals experience more intimacy with their pets than they have ever done with a human. Perhaps all this is inevitable in a society that subtly discourages touching between humans and where so many people have no one with whom to be intimate.

Even this is not the whole story, however, because a few people find that they can be intimate only with inanimate objects. As we saw on page 10 this is probably healthy in the context of 'being at one with the cosmos' yet if this is our only source of intimacy there is usually something wrong. Early in life babies and toddlers who have insufficient loving attention from their care-giver often turn to objects as love substitutes. The security blankets, rags, teddies or pacifiers that many such children carry around with them are known, in psychological jargon, as transitional objects. These represent, in an almost magical way, the absent parent and its attendant love and intimacy. A baby's dummy or pacifier can become a real source of physical intimacy in the absence of its mother's nipple. In later life we suck pencils, smoke pipes and cigarettes, chew on spectacle ends, chew gum, and so on. This is reminiscent of old oral pleasures and intimacies and usually shows that we had too little oral intimacy when we really needed it.

All sorts of jewellery, clothing, bedclothes, furniture and other objects can be caressed or used to caress us. A bath full of warm water can feel womb-like at both the conscious and unconscious level. Clothing touches our bodies in a way that is highly intimate. When working on this subject with a woman I often find that progress dramatically occurs when she finds she wants to buy more sensual underwear. This tiny but significant first step can be the initial evidence that she is starting to 'make love' to her own body as a prelude to incorporating her lover in her physical intimacies. Sex toys – from pop posters to inflatable rubber dolls – are all objects with which people can be sexually intimate. These contrast starkly with the other, highly symbolic sexual things we have looked at here.

In an ideal world in which our basic intimacy needs were adequately met in infancy and childhood, most such substitutes would be redundant. The fact is, however, that most of us have far from perfect experiences of intimacy; in our formative years some of us have very harmful ones. The human craving for physical intimacy seeks out other channels of expression and whole industries have sprung up to satisfy these primitive longings. Until the very nature of parenting changes in our culture millions of people will continue to seek the physical and even emotional intimacy they need in ways that largely exclude other humans. This was, after all, their experience early in life and they are simply repeating it.

Trouble brews when we start to address the question of whether we should, for example, be kissing our beloved rather than smoking a cigarette. I have no answers to this, if only because no single human being can cater for all our needs for physical intimacy even if we elect to restrict the expression of genital intimacy to him or her alone. So even the most loved and intimate individual might still enjoy the tactile sensations of a comfy chair or a cigar. It seems to me that problems could be said to occur when the balance between intimacy expressed as part of an interpersonal relationship and that with other 'objects', animate or inanimate, causes a disturbance in the individual's life. At various stages of life we express our intimacy needs in different ways. A little child might be highly intimate with his or her teddy bear; an adult with his or her partner; and an elderly single person with his or her pet. Who would care to say which of these is most valid?

Physical intimacy in all its forms appears to be vital to human beings from the cradle onwards. Whether or not we get what we need from the earliest days of life colours how we view such intimacy throughout our lives. Good experiences early on set us up for all our physically intimate dealings with friends and lovers, whether we simply want to hug those we love as a sign of affection or seek much deeper physical connection in the uniqueness of sexual intercourse. Adverse events, even those often repeated throughout childhood, need not necessarily spell disaster for our future intimate life, though if we have a largely negative background in this respect we are at further risk when it comes to choosing a partner for life. Being aware of our past hurts helps us in selecting such a partner and helps prevent us from falling into the same traps. I hope that anyone who has read even this far will be better equipped to avoid some of the more obvious pitfalls.

Physical intimacy, as we have seen, rarely stands alone in human dealings, especially close and meaningful ones between lovers. This makes such physical business very important, even if genital activity is poor or non-existent. The elderly, the single, the mentally disadvantaged, the terminally ill, the sick and the lonely all have their physical needs for intimacy with or without genital connection, yet in our culture we all too often ignore such needs. It is not only the young, the healthy and the beautiful who have a right to experience intimacy.

Transforming everything in Parts One and Two of this book from theory into practice is not easy. It takes knowledge, effort and goodwill. Part Three now deals with the practical work involved in this transformation.

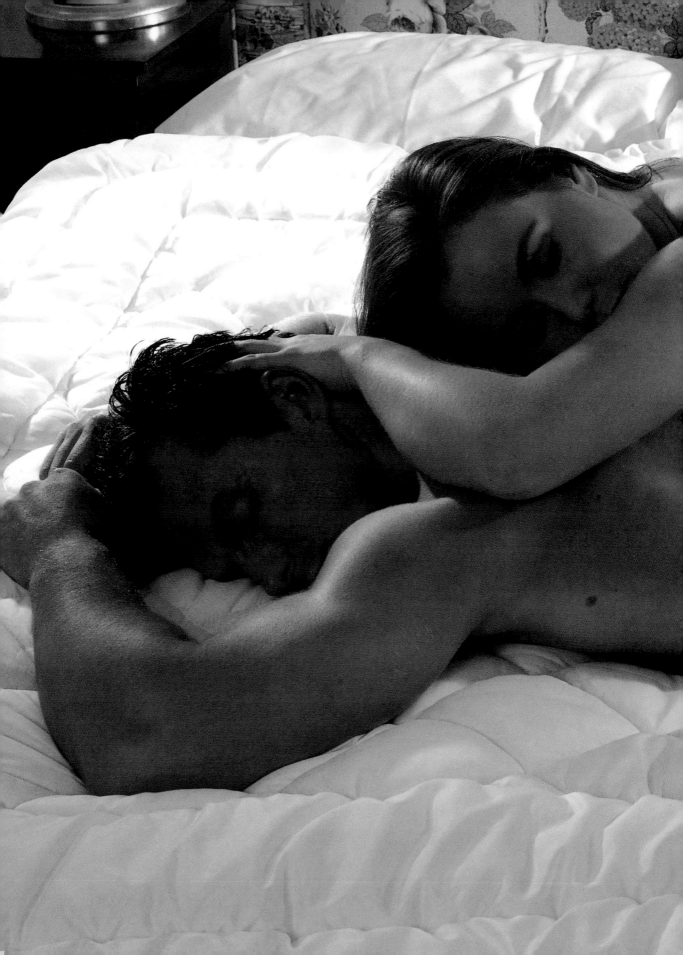

BUILDING YOUR INTIMATE LIFE

No matter how much two people love one another or know the theory nothing happens by magic to make them more intimate. In this section we look at some of the practical ways that I use to help people learn the art and craft of intimacy. I use the phrase 'art and craft' advisedly because not only do our heart, intuition and soul play a part in our intimate life but so too do all kinds of learned behaviours and skills. This part of the book addresses all of these areas.

Only a foolish individual would claim with any certainty where to embark on the journey towards a deeper and more intimate relationship. In this section, I have gathered together some of the many and varied pieces of 'homework' that I have used in my work with couples over the years.

We often have a laugh about doing this homework and frequently one or other partner quite openly questions the value or even the validity of a particular task I have set. Almost without exception, though, he or she has a change of heart once time and love really start to be invested in the exercise concerned and the most sceptical individual often ends up getting the most out of the task in question.

When I work on the development of intimacy in therapy with a couple I tailor-make a one-off plan for them, starting where we all agree they are at the time and building week by week from there. This is, however, not possible in a book because I cannot know at what stage my readers are in their intimate relationships.

What I suggest you do is to start at the beginning and go through all of the exercises, if only because even if you think you know it all or have no problems in that particular area I can promise you that you will gain a lot more than you ever imagined. Try to remain open to the possibility that any of us could benefit from each and every one of these exercises, whatever the stage of our relationship. We simply embark on the journey of discovery from where we are at the time. It is also fun and instructive to return to the very same activity some years later and see how far you have come. Couples often tell me that when they do this they are astonished that they see the same topic from a completely new angle. It is as if they have new spectacles.

Please do not look at the exercises and panic. It is easy to take fright at the enormity of the task. In practice, I never lay out everything like this on day one. In this way my patients cannot see what I have planned for them and give up in horror. How about taking each exercise one at a time and simply progressing gently on to the next as and when you have the time and energy to do so? There is no rush to dash through them. Take your time. You may find that one particular exercise takes you by surprise and that it will take a lot of time before you can feel sufficiently confident to go on to the next. On other occasions you will both be happy to romp through several in one week.

Do not forget also that it is a *relationship* you are dealing with and that when doing this sort of task together it helps to remember that our partner may not be able, or willing, to proceed at our pace. This can be annoying at times, but any individual sufficiently interested in making his or her relationship more intimate will be prepared to wait for the other to 'catch up'. The Ancient Orientals had a lovely phrase for this: 'Take your tiger to the mountain'. This is what we all have to do in any relationship that is growing and changing. The one who is waiting has to take his or her tiger to the mountain while the other comes to meet them. This waiting can often be very painful and calls for the utmost love and patience. But the waiting is always worthwhile both for the one who waits (because soon it will be his or her turn to be struggling while the other waits) and for the one who is working hard to change and grow (because of the knowledge that his or her beloved is there).

It is always difficult to know what to call the sorts of task or activity that I am suggesting in this part of the book. I have settled on the term 'exercise' because although it sounds rather like school work it does have the advantage of describing exactly what is involved. None of the homework described here can ever truly be said to be completed because wherever we are in our relationship we can start from there and build and learn from even the simplest task. Just as physical exercise tones up the body these tasks keep us sexually and emotionally 'fit', however expert or able we think we are.

This is an important concept in the growth and maintenance of intimacy. Just as a concert pianist still practises his scales every day, as a beginner does, so too should we all do the same type of work on our loving life together. As with any form of *physical* exercise, repetition makes it easier to do and the level of fitness obtained is all the more rewarding. So it is with these tasks. They are not ends in themselves as some who seek to ridicule such activities assert; they cannot by themselves create a more intimate relationship; but the time, dedication, effort, energy and loving investment they call for help develop any relationship. In this sense lessons learned here can be transferred to other parts of our lives within our family or at work. Many individuals have told me that this kind of investment in themselves and their relationship has yielded a rich harvest in their working lives, often leading to promotion as others around them perceive the increased empathy and intimacy of which they are capable.

How you use this section will be up to you. If you are starting out together as a young couple or even in middle age for the second time around then perhaps it would make sense to go through all the steps one at a time, not progressing on to the next until you are completely happy with where you are. Most readers, however, will not be at this stage of their love lives. Perhaps, then, the best way to use this part of the book is to take a section you think will benefit you and your partner and to complete it to your joint satisfaction. Jump around various parts selecting those sections that you think most apply. Even if you decide to take this 'choosing from the menu' approach, try out a section from time to time that you think you can do pretty easily. You could be surprised how much you will learn even if you think your relationship is already good. In fact, as many couples have told me, some of the most simple-sounding parts of this programme yield the most astonishing results if they are approached with sincerity and an open mind.

Working towards intimacy is a lifelong task. The most important and difficult single skill required is to be able to focus on ourselves. When couples come to me to start dealing with their intimacy problems they are almost invariably 'other-focused'. They can see the other person's problems and faults very clearly and inform me and their partner that everything would be fine if only the other would change. This approach takes us nowhere. The only person we can change is ourself and until we can put at least some of the energy we spend focusing on our partner to work on ourselves we end up going around in circles.

You will find that you will get the best out of this book if you really try to understand the principles that underly the exercises in this section. Simply 'doing things better' is not enough. Techniques and skills never in themselves provide answers;

they have to be based on a solid understanding at head and heart level. There are no quick fixes when it comes to building an intimate life and as you work through this section you will soon see how challenging it is as the complexities and ambiguities arise and crave a solution.

Expect, also, quite a lot of resistance from within yourself and your partner. This will almost certainly come from the unconscious and will not be 'deliberate'. As we seek to change to become more intimate all kinds of unconscious circuits assert themselves and do their best to make our task difficult. If this occurs you will know you are on the right track and that you are challenging your defences. Patience, love and perseverance will usually bring the results you want.

When I say that we need to become self-focused I do not mean that we should start to blame ourselves for everything. This is no call for remaining in a victim role, the butt of unfairness or injustice. The sort of self-focusing I have in mind is that which forces us to take personal responsibility for the things we can and should change about ourselves. It also goes a step further than simply acknowledging that we cannot and should not seek to change our partner; it brings a state of humility that admits just how little we can ever know about people in general and our partner in particular. So many people I see work on the 'I know what is best for you' principle with their partner and it is clear that this is dangerous in maintaining old pathological states.

As we take the spotlight off our partner and focus it on ourselves we become less of an expert on him or her and more informed about ourselves. Now our feedback to our partner starts to be really useful as we resist our knee-jerk responses and other-centredness. This is very hard for rescuers (see page 52) who may have spent a lifetime focusing on others to protect themselves from their own pain but it is hugely rewarding emotionally and brings good results practically. Such change does not happen overnight, though. Our partner will have to come to trust our new, self-aware position before he or she, in turn, can make reciprocal changes. As we start on our journey of self-awareness we take a much more responsible position in the relationship based on our own values, beliefs and principles rather than as some sort of reaction to how our partner defines the relationship. This autonomy brings meaningful intimacy, contrary to what almost everyone starting out thinks will be the case.

Perhaps the biggest hurdle that people erect when I start to suggest all this is their fear of losing the relationship. 'If I really start to be me, as I truly am, will he/she like me, want me, or love me?' is the sort of emotion that soon raises its head. I have pointed out to individuals countless times that there is a fundamental paradox in all this: *we cannot begin our journey towards real intimacy until we can convince ourselves that we can live without the relationship.* Taking risks is a vital part of the process and the individual who is unwilling or unable to do so will find the path long and hard or even impossible. This makes for difficulties when trying to grow as a couple because one of us will almost certainly be further along the track of self-focusing and readiness to put the relationship on the line than the other. There is no easy answer except to start from where you each are and to acknowledge your different starting points.

—————— EXERCISE ONE ——————

WHY CAN'T YOU HEAR WHAT I'M SAYING?

I make no apologies for starting off with a very difficult challenge. By mastering this skill early on you will find it much easier to tackle all the other exercises you will be doing over the weeks or months it takes you to lay the foundations of your new intimate life.

One thing that people, women especially, endlessly complain about is that their partner does not understand them. More to the point, perhaps, that they do not *feel* understood. This usually means that they are not being listened to in an empathic way.

Before we actually begin this listening exercise, let us start by seeing what empathy is. First of all, it *is not* sympathy. When I first start doing this exercise with couples in the consulting room, one or other says something like 'I know exactly how you feel' and then recounts something from his or her present or past experiences that illustrates how well he or she is placed to understand what the other is saying or feeling. This sympathetic approach in which the listener mirrors from personal experience what he or she hears *can* be useful later on but for now *do not do it*.

Empathy is different from sympathy in that when I am being empathic with you I put my own business to one side and put myself in your shoes. By doing so I can, if only for a moment or two, feel *with* you what it is that you are feeling. I cannot and would not wish to feel your feelings for you: they are yours, not mine. But with empathy I can get into your skin and identify with you very deeply.

However, there are no prizes for being able to do this simply so that we can say, 'I know exactly what Jill is feeling – I'm really in there with her.' Good though this might make *me* feel it does little or nothing for Jill. The secret of good empathic listening is to respond to our partner and his or her feelings in such a way that he or she *knows* that we have heard and have identified the feelings correctly. This is the first and most important step to feeling understood and lays the best possible foundation for all the intimacy work in this part of the book.

Now let us look at the three main aspects of empathic listening in more detail, and work through some ways of improving skills in this fundamentally important area.

The first thing to do is to put your own ego to one side. Do not jump in with *your* business. Try to block out all *your* thoughts and feelings about the topic under discussion and listen solely to your partner. This can be the most difficult part of empathic listening because in our culture we are all brought up to be ego-centred, to put the 'I' first. Unhooking from this can be a major task, especially for men. With love and practice, though, you will be surprised how quickly you can lose your bad habits, if you really want to. And wanting to is the secret because none of this is easy, especially early on.

When it actually comes to putting our ego to one side in order to listen empathically there are many roadblocks or obstacles to success. Some of the more common ones are listed here. See which apply to you, whether it be all of the time or just occasionally, and make some conscious efforts to stop them, perhaps with the help of your partner.

- I am preoccupied.
- I am working out what to say next.
- My feelings are too strong (about what I hear or about something else).
- I do not like the content or feelings of what I hear and so I am denying/rejecting/ignoring it.
- What I hear triggers words or ideas that make me uncomfortable.
- I try to rescue others through reassurance.
- My arrogance makes others believe that their thoughts/feelings are insignificant/worthless.
- I show too much concern
- I compete for attention by talking about my own experience.
- My insecurity makes me need to justify or defend myself.
- I silently criticize/evaluate/find fault.
- I advise/control/lead/direct.
- I interrupt.
- I read too deeply into what is said.
- I do not notice mixed messages: the body language not matching what is being said.
- I am impatient (the other's fear of not being heard leads to a sort of 'verbal clinging', which increases my impatience).
- I am curious so I question/interrogate.

Continued on page 132

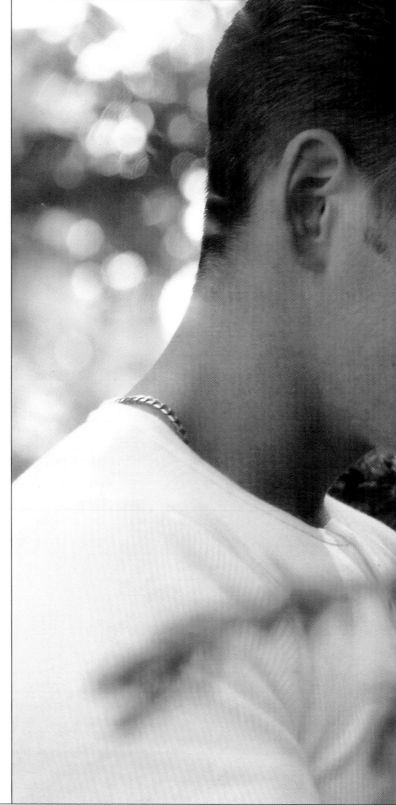

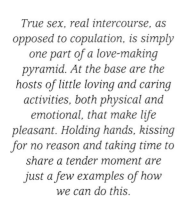

True sex, real intercourse, as opposed to copulation, is simply one part of a love-making pyramid. At the base are the hosts of little loving and caring activities, both physical and emotional, that make life pleasant. Holding hands, kissing for no reason and taking time to share a tender moment are just a few examples of how we can do this.

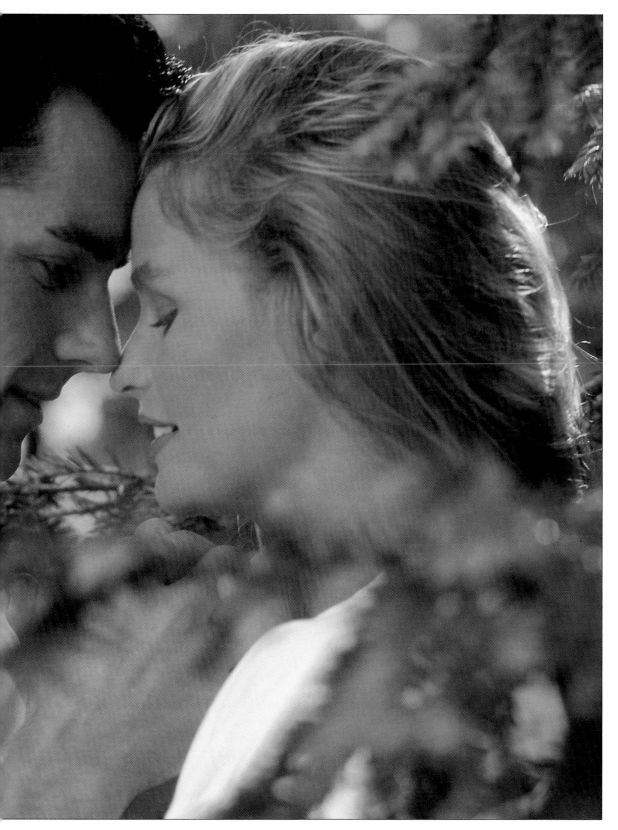

- I think I know what the other will say because I have heard it before or know this person so well (I already know what you are going to say so I will interpret everything you say in the light of this 'knowledge' and make assumptions).
- I race ahead of the speaker in my thinking.
- I jump to premature conclusions.
- I stereotype the speaker and what is said.
- I dismiss what is said because I do not like the speaker, what he or she stands for or has done.
- I fill silences that make me feel uncomfortable.
- I have never made an effort to listen.
- I want to punish/put down the speaker by not listening.
- The speaker hits one of my 'no-go areas' (see page 151).

Always remember that your own emotional neediness, either in the present or from the past, will sometimes preclude you from listening skilfully. It helps if you can recognize and act on this, particularly when you are feeling fraught.

The second essential part of empathic listening involves identifying your partner's main feelings as he or she talks. This is relatively easy if the feelings are big and obvious, such as anger, rage, fear, joy or helplessness. It may be much more difficult, however, if they are 'softer' emotions, such as doubt, confusion, satisfaction or happiness.

I find that many couples have great difficulty when it comes to identifying emotions. Just being asked to name some emotions can cause problems. The following list of common feelings might help you to become more aware of what your partner could be expressing.

sadness	doubt	friendliness
misery	humiliation	joy
isolation	inadequacy	love
rejection	shyness	affection
unlovability	embarrassment	caring
unworthiness	exhaustion	confidence
hopelessness	boredom	interest
disappointment	fury	relaxation
betrayal	loneliness	relief
irritability	warmth	surprise
apprehension	pleasure	thankfulness
'madness'	arousal	importance
disgust	comfort	certainty
shock	tenderness	determination

As you can see there are scores of possible emotions that we can pick up if we are sufficiently skilled. The secret is to learn how to discern exactly what our partner *is* feeling and this can be tricky. In order to get it anywhere near right we have to be aware of body language; the tone and quality of voice; the context in which all of this is occurring; what our partner is actually saying; and what he or she *appears* to be saying. If you have not yet read the section concerning feelings and metafeelings (see page 29) it could be helpful to do so now.

The third important skill involved in empathic listening is being able to reflect the feelings you have perceived back to your partner so that he or she feels understood. This sounds terribly corny at first but try saying something like, 'It seems to me you're feeling . . .'. If you are right, and you may or may not be early on, then your partner will agree with you and will feel pleased that he or she has been heard and understood. The beauty of this type of 'open-ended' communication style is that I have yet to come across anybody who, having had their feelings reflected in this way, shuts up and walks off. Quite the contrary. What usually happens is that the speaker immediately follows up with another statement, often one that shares something really important to him or her. In this way what could have easily become a dead-end conversation now opens up to be really useful as the speaker feels heard, not just by your ears but by your heart and soul as well. This is the start of intimate communication and makes both parties feel better.

If you happen to name the wrong emotion your partner can tell you so and you will learn that that particular combination of body language, emotional expression and speech means something else in your partner's case. This is real learning worth its weight in gold because it enables us to personalize our emotional knowledge of our partner and to stop jumping to conclusions based on our experience of others in similar situations. Perhaps an example will help show how this works. Jim comes home from work one evening feeling wretched. 'That Paul will have to go, he'll be the death of me!' I'll sack him next week if he does that again.' His wife, having had a bad day with the kids and feeling totally unempathic retorts, 'You think *you've* got problems. I've had a hell of a day. The washing-machine leaked and Johnny has a terrible cold.' Jim looks disbelievingly at her. He has not been heard. His emotions have not been acknowledged and he goes off in a huff, wounded and silent. Neither Jim nor his wife feel understood, both feel hurt, they do not have sex that night – another nail in their sexual coffin.

How much better if his wife had responded empathically by saying something like; 'I can see you're really frustrated about Paul. He seems to make your life hell at the moment.' Whether or not this were accompanied by even the tiniest physical sign of affection they would have shared a real moment of intimacy and their lives would have come closer together. My experience is that instead of going off to the pub or slumping down in front of the TV such a man quickly starts to engage in his wife's emotional business and listens to her about *her* day. In this way both feel understood and loved and their love life gains hugely *because* of life's unavoidable pains and traumas rather than *in spite of* them. We all have problems and traumas in life. Intimate couples, though, differ from most others in that they acknowledge this as a reality and help one another get through them. They do not compete for time and space on the emotional stage because they know from experience that they will each have sufficient of both.

The sort of listening we have looked at in this exercise – listening and being heard from the heart – is the start of all intimate dealings on a practical basis day by day. Nowhere is this more important than when we are trying to hear one another on matters to do with sex and romance. I work on the general principle that the most difficult areas of all on which to communicate are those where there is a high level of unconscious activity. Sex rates about the highest on this scale.

All of this means that unless we can truly listen to one another in this way we will not stand much chance of building an intimate life together. This is why I have, and always do, put this exercise first. But do not be fooled into thinking that this comes easily. It does not. It can take weeks or months of practice at putting your own ego to one side, identifying emotions and reflecting back to your partner what you have perceived. Most people find that this works best if they practise this sort of listening in everyday life first and then come to their partner with their skills at least somewhat honed. It is an almost universal experience that the person to whom it is most difficult to listen empathically is our loved partner.

WHY CAN'T YOU BE MORE LIKE ME?

The vast majority of us work on the assumption that we are normal and therefore right. This having to be right is a major barrier to intimacy (see page 80) but we cannot blame ourselves for feeling this way because most of us have never really explored how different we are as individuals in our partnership. We saw why and how opposites attract on page 35 but here let us look at a useful piece of homework that you can do together. This, like most of the exercises, will probably provide seedcorn for many conversations.

We all come to our partnership with attitudes, both conscious and unconscious, lifted directly and unexamined from our family of origin. It makes sense, therefore, to air these so that we can make them real to one another and start accepting each other *for* our differences rather than punishing our partner, however unwittingly, for not being like us.

Take a sheet of paper each and write the following topics down the left-hand side: money; sex; work; fun; religion; food; education; family; friends; the role of women; the role of men. On the right, make a few notes about what your family thought and felt about these subjects. Go for knee-jerk responses and write the first thing that comes to your mind. Do not try to be clever, and certainly do not write a PhD on the subject. The topics I have suggested are to start you off and you will probably want to add your own.

Once you have completed your comments about each topic, exchange sheets and read your partner's carefully. Use this as a way of opening up a conversation about the differences between your families. Remember that neither of you is right and that you are *both* right. An interesting addition to this exercise is to write down what your (usually unspoken) family motto was. Compare notes and see how these mottos affect your life together today.

We are the product of all our yesterdays, as we have seen. Understanding the family baggage we carry with us and trying hard to accept that we are different but alright can not only be highly illuminating to our partner but also a vital building block in creating intimacy.

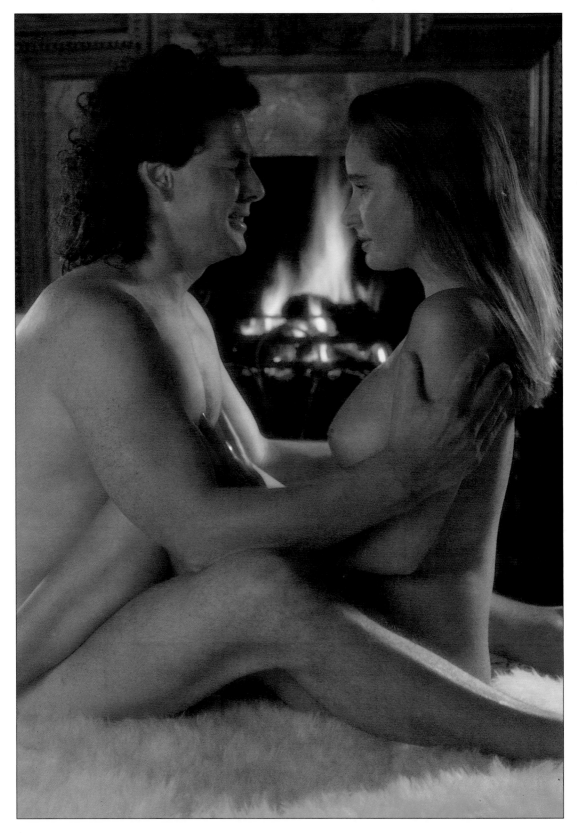

---EXERCISE THREE---

HOW SATISFIED ARE YOU?

The way we see our intimate relationship can be different from the way our partner sees it and satisfaction levels vary hugely. So long as the balance is fairly equal all is well. If one of us feels less benefited, however, things start to go wrong. Sex is usually the first casualty.

In my experience, couples working towards a more intimate relationship can benefit from carrying out an 'audit' of their relationship, even at this relatively early stage in the process. Finding out about how satisfied we and our partner are with specific areas of the relationship can be greatly beneficial in the move towards intimacy. This exercise is designed to help you do this.

Draw up a list together of subjects that you wish to discuss. Here are some examples: intimacy, sex, children, money, jobs, family life, holidays, friendship, hobbies, recreation, decision-making, resolving conflict. Add your own items that personalize the list to your partnership. Go through the list separately from each other (each with your own sheet of paper). Give each of the topics a score out of five for how satisfied you are with them today.

Sharing with one another the areas of life that satisfy you most and least gives you an opportunity to help one another build up the low-scoring areas and take a delight in the high-scoring ones. The most valuable part of this exercise is not the scores themselves but the different perceptions that surface about the same topic. This can be a source of considerable intimacy whether you agree or disagree and links in well with Exercise Two, which is about accepting difference.

Amy might say, for example, that she feels very financially secure in her marriage and so give this topic a score of five. Ben, however, might give it only one point. Sharing these very different perceptions of the same matter is part of the nitty-gritty of actually living an intimate life rather than simply theorizing about it.

A memorable encounter, such as this kind of love-making session, not only gives us a yardstick by which to measure other intimate moments but can also feed our fantasy life.

---EXERCISE FOUR---

WHAT IS THE MOST INTIMATE YOU HAVE EVER FELT?

Sit down one day with your partner and jot down on a piece of paper the answers to three questions: 1) What is the most intimate you have ever felt; with whom; and when? 2) How do you know you feel intimate with someone (not necessarily your partner)? 3) How would you most like your partner to be intimate with you? Having read the book this far you should have plenty of ideas.

This can be a tricky exercise because it begins to focus on shortcomings in a way that may be taken personally by your partner. Men especially tend to react badly, fearing that any criticism about the present or the revelation that their partner felt more intimate with a past lover, mother, colleague or whomever, implies that they are useless. A vital part of becoming truly intimate is being able to accept this sort of reality for what it is – a starting point for growth and change – not a damning criticism or a character assassination. Only by reflecting on those relationships in our lives that have really felt intimate can we hope to create anything equally or more rewarding with our partner. The individual who is unwilling to learn from such an exploration cannot hope to live a realistic life with his or her mate and intimacy as I define it will be impossible.

---EXERCISE FIVE---

HOW DO YOU SABOTAGE YOUR INTIMATE RELATIONSHIP?

Most people claim to have too little intimacy in their lives. The vast majority of us, however, are busy unconsciously sabotaging our chances, even when we have people around us who are capable of being intimate with us.

How do *you* do this? Make some time for yourself and think this through. Do you constantly test your relationship, perhaps to destruction? Do you have unrealistic expectations? Do you unwittingly avoid your partner? Do you invest enough time in your relationship? How much energy do you devote to its maintenance? Do you secretly fear success and the changes that real intimacy will bring to your life-style? And so on.

Next think about how your partner consciously or unconsciously sabotages your intimate relationship. What could you do to ensure that this happens less frequently? Given that you can change only yourself, work out some ways of dealing with your partner's sabotage techniques.

On another occasion get together and share what you have discovered. The vast majority of us shoot our intimate lives in the foot quite unconsciously and it can often be useful and enlightening to listen to our partner, or even to someone else who loves us, as they are frequently more able than we are ourselves to put their finger on the ways in which we sabotage that which we claim we most want.

EXERCISE SIX

HOW DO YOU KNOW YOU ARE NOT GETTING ENOUGH INTIMACY?

Many, if not most of those who complain to me that their lives lack intimacy, are unaware how it is that they manifest this lack. If we *are* aware of what is going on in this respect then not only can we begin to make sense of all kinds of previously inexplicable events and experiences in our lives, but also our partner can read us better and, hopefully, help us to help ourselves in this difficult area of life.

People seem to manifest their lack of intimacy in three ways: physically, emotionally and behaviourally. As a therapist who puts considerable emphasis on the body and what it has to teach us, I often start with the body when working on these matters with an individual or a couple. Some people I see, for example, have endless headaches (which they usually call migraines); others have sexual problems; others bowel or intestinal ailments; some women experience repeated cystitis; other individuals have trouble keeping their blood pressure down, even with drugs, and so on. The bodies of all of these people are telling them something about their innermost emotional and spiritual state. Often the most remarkable healing can occur as the individual experiences true intimacy, perhaps for the first time in his or her life.

Emotional problems such as depression, anxiety, mood swings, helplessness and hopelessness can also be ways in which we show our lack of intimacy. In my deepest analytical work with people who react in this way to a lack of intimacy I usually find that adverse baby and childhood experiences lie at the heart of their problem. Many such people have never experienced real intimacy in their lives and unconsciously choose a partner who will continue this hurtful model.

Lastly, and very commonly, we can express our lack of intimacy in behavioural ways. Some of the most frequently encountered are smoking, excessive drinking, weight-control problems, binge eating, gambling, compulsive dating or sex, repeated driving offences, and so on. Many such compulsive and repetitive types of behaviour stem from too little intimacy at some stage in life and can be the bolt-hole that we run to as a way of propping ourselves up when we cannot obtain the intimacy we so crave.

I am not suggesting that all the problems I have listed in this exercise can be healed by increasing the amount of intimacy in our lives, but it always helps. Often it can make a massive difference. Perhaps most important is for a couple to understand one another well enough and to be sufficiently accepting of one another's underlying woundedness to be able to deal lovingly with these sorts of behaviour. Rather than punishing our partner, being compassionate and empathic will enable the sufferer to feel heard, loved and accepted in spite of, or even because of his or her problems. This, in turn, enables our partner to experience intimacy in a healing way. Even people who have what I call a medical 'plumbing' problem – something that is wrong with the nuts and bolts of their bodies – say that increased levels of intimacy in their relationship often make them feel better, sometimes after many years of suffering with a physical ailment that has resisted treatment.

Make all this the subject of one of your talks. By becoming more aware of how both of you show your lack of intimacy, you will be better able to make allowances. You will probably notice tangible improvements as you work through this programme of exercises over some weeks or months.

EXERCISE SEVEN

IS GIVING MORE NOBLE THAN RECEIVING?

There are very few relationships in any area of life in which both partners find it equally easy to give and receive. Some people are brought up to be 'givers', or perhaps more insidiously 'rescuers' (see page 52). Understandably they carry this model with them and act it out in their adult partnerships.

Working together towards greater intimacy is probably the most coequal job you will ever have done in your life as a couple. As I have repeatedly pointed out, no one is right and no one wrong in this task. When one of us is a natural giver or rescuer, however, it immediately puts the other in danger of becoming a poor little 'victim' who is being 'done good to'. This is the antithesis of intimacy and is certain to wreck your efforts in no time at all.

Take some time to assess the balance of giving and receiving in your relationship. (You will probably find that one of you is more of a giver and the other is more of a receiver.) The amount of giving and receiving you both do will, however, vary according to the matter in hand. Go through a list of areas that affect your life together and try to appraise honestly which of you does most giving or receiving in each of the settings. Then discuss how this is helpful (or not as the case may be) to you and your journey towards intimacy. Use the following as a starting list but, as always, add your own items to personalize it to your relationship: money; affection; humour; presents; trust; sex; praise; respect; space; apologies; forgiveness; promises; commitment; touch.

Some females in our culture take control of the emotional giving in a relationship, for example. This can be fine but often works to their disadvantage because their man then sees himself as shut out or even as totally inept in this area of life. Many's the man who has told me that given 'permission' from me he has found it easy, rewarding and valuable to his relationship to be much more emotionally giving. Sometimes, however, the wife, whose domain this has previously been, complains that he is treading on 'her territory'. This comes as hugely ironic, and we often have a laugh about it, because the very same woman not two weeks before has often complained bitterly that she is married to an emotional cripple.

EXERCISE EIGHT

WHAT DO YOU THINK YOU WANT?

By this stage you should be getting some firm ideas about what you want from an intimate relationship so this is a good time to think about your expectations. As with almost everything to do with our loving and sexual lives our expectations go before us, often laying a minefield in which we are almost bound to lose the odd foot or two. By now you should both be realistic enough to set out the parameters that seem important to you as individuals. Remember the 'difference' exercise when doing this (see page 133). There is no point in coming this far only to say in amazement, as many of my couples do, 'You must be joking! I wouldn't call that intimate at all.'

The following list suggests some of the areas you might like to consider when trying to define *your* idea of a really intimate life with your lover.

- Sharing political views.
- Working together.
- Having/not having children.
- Making love beautifully.
- Having the same spiritual or religious views.
- Talking to one another about deep matters.
- Communicating easily on a day-to-day basis.
- Being sexually faithful.
- Being best friends.
- Being good parents.
- Sharing hobbies.

Begin by looking at one another's list and seeing what you agree on. Make a fresh list of these items. Next, check off the things that look very difficult and agree to leave these for a while. Then create a list of the items that you *could* work on jointly.

Continued on page 140

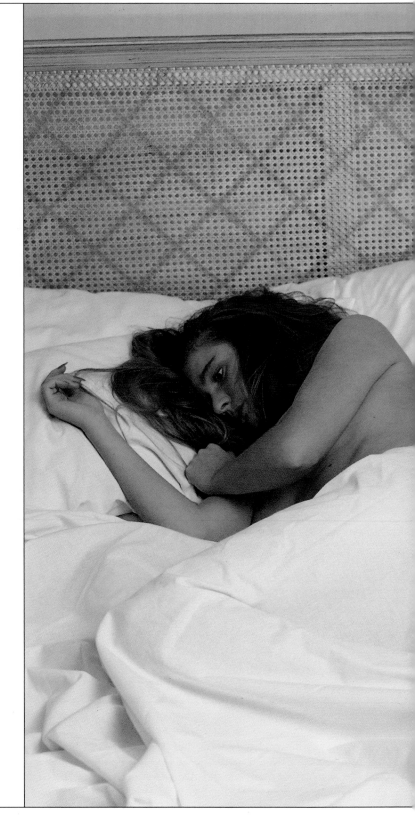

Failure is an inevitable part of any intimate couple's experience. The very act of experimenting, trying to change and being more intimate involves taking risks. This can lead to the occasional 'failure' and let-down but the truly intimate couple can usually overcome such hurdles as they draw on the store of goodwill and understanding that they have built up over the years.

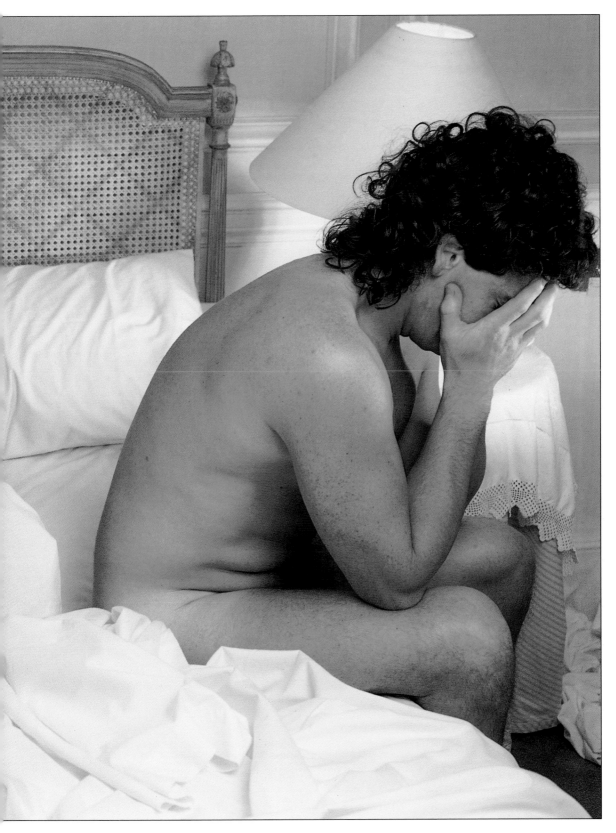

Now comes the difficult part. This entails taking three of the items from each of your lists and agreeing that over the next week you will really try to make something good happen for your partner in each of the three areas. Let us say, for example, that Penny says that her three areas would be: 1) having her hand held while out in a public place, such as shopping; 2) being listened to for two minutes as she talks about her day at work; and 3) being shown the bank statements when they arrive. Her partner would then make it his priority to ensure that these things were done in a way that was meaningful *to her* at least once in the following week. She, in turn, undertakes to do the same for and with him on *his* important intimacy issues.

This is an excellent exercise because it shows that we accept our lover and his or her needs and that we are prepared to alter our behaviour to make our partner feel what he or she considers intimate. It works wonders.

———————— EXERCISE NINE ————————

WHEN DID YOU LAST COURT ONE ANOTHER?

Many couples I see consider courtship a quaint concept that went out with the Ark. They feel that it is somehow immature or adolescent and definitely not a behaviour that should be continued within a long-term relationship. Nothing could be further from the truth. Courtship is the gracious, loving behaviour we show to our partner that makes him or her feel special in a romantic way. It is certainly true that most of us engage in at least some of this when we first start going out together, but my clinical experience shows that most couples soon give it up in favour of 'real sex'. Usually, but by no means always, this move comes from the man.

The first stage of this exercise is to look at your relationship and to see what you are already doing that *is* romantic and could be called courtship behaviour. Try to complete the following sentence by filling in a behaviour that is unique to you as a pair of *lovers*. 'I feel really loved and special in our relationship when you . . .' This is different from looking at existing types of intimate behaviour in your relationship

because, frankly, those items, or many of them, could apply to any intimate relationship: between two really close friends or between a parent and child, for example.

Here are some examples of courtship behaviour to get your discussions under way. Remember that you may well have rather different definitions of what constitutes courtship behaviour:

- Phoning me at the office just to say you love me.
- Giving and receiving little presents 'for no reason'.
- Massaging my shoulders when I come in from work exhausted.
- Giving me a peck on the cheek in public.
- Caressing or holding me in a way that neither of us expects to end in sex.
- Behaving courteously to me in social matters.
- Writing love letters or poetry to me.
- Reading to me.
- Buying me flowers.
- Making it plain to others that we are 'a unit' – special and deeply involved.

Now think back to the courtship behaviours you *used* to enjoy as a couple and make a list of these.

Next exchange lists and agree on three items that you could start doing with ease. As with Exercise Eight, try to make these happen as frequently as you can or is practical. Over some weeks you will find that you slowly build up a bank of courtship behaviour and that at least some of these practices will start to become second nature. These in themselves will not assure you of a more intimate life together, but taken as a whole with all the other exercises they start to create an encouraging base for more sexual intimacy. Most women who have complaints in this area of their relationship tell me that they see 'foreplay' as starting as soon as they get up in the morning, not ten minutes before their man wants to penetrate them later that evening.

———————————————————

Some people unwisely think of courtship as an outdated and rather silly practice in which to indulge once past their teens. Yet most people, especially women, say that courtship rituals are important throughout their life with their partner.

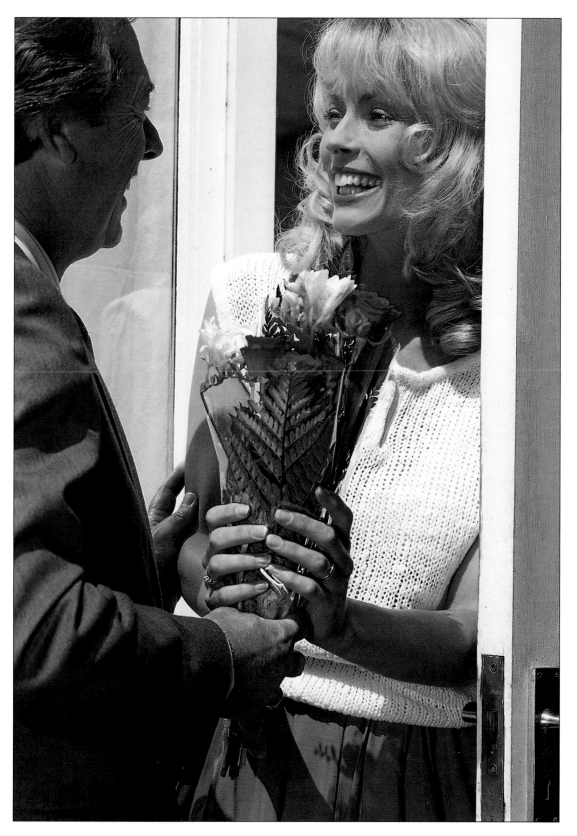

—————————— EXERCISE TEN ——————————

DO WE HAVE TO 'HAVE SEX' ALL THE TIME OR COULD WE TRY TO MAKE LOVE?

So far I have hardly mentioned sex. I have done this advisedly. Although many couples come to me because their sex life is a disaster and their intimate life much the same, I almost never achieve any results unless we first deal with the sorts of issues I have outlined in Exercises One to Nine. Sometimes one or other partner insists that I get on to the 'real' business: better sex. In retrospect, however, almost everyone agrees that to go for an improvement in sex before dealing with intimacy is to put the cart before the horse.

Without wishing to sound too mechanical, the journey from 'having sex' or 'copulating' to making love is not one that can be negotiated at one leap, even if you have already come this far and have built a truly intimate relationship. All the effort you have made will yield dividends but simply *hoping* that this alone will lead to a great sex life is not enough. As you embark on this stage of your growth towards sexual intimacy please do not forget to keep up any good lessons you have learned and rewarding behaviours that have now become a part of your loving and non-genital life together.

There are ten steps that I use to guide couples from 'sex' to love-making. Let us look at each in turn. Take your time, as with the other exercises and discuss your thoughts and feelings with one another using all your new-found skills.

STEP ONE: GET TO KNOW YOUR OWN BODY AND GENITALS

When starting on our journey to greater sexual intimacy it is vital to set off from the right place. Many individuals I see criticize their partner for not being physically or sexually intimate with them, yet have not realized that their partner is unconsciously picking up messages that say 'I am not happy being intimate with myself' and so backs off.

The place to begin, then, is to get to know your own body. Do this alone in front of a mirror. Look at what you see and try to accept the good with the bad. You almost certainly will not have a perfect figure and look like the people in advertisements but try to be realistic about what your good features are and to accept with some grace the things you cannot change. Having said this, there may well be things you *can* change. You may be overweight for example; you may have let yourself go bodily and need to take some exercise to tone yourself up; your fingers may be stained with nicotine; your nails tatty; and so on. Many such items of personal appearance can be altered given the will.

At this stage the task is, therefore, to get to know your naked body and to start on the process of getting to like it. When in the bath, close your eyes and massage yourself, finding out where feels nicest. Out of the bath, take the phone off the hook, ensure that you are private, get the room warm and slowly and gently explore your body all over (except for your genitals) to find out what feels best to you. I usually suggest giving each anatomical area a score out of five where five is the best you can possibly imagine. Over several sessions you should be able to build up a sensuality profile of your own body and you may well be surprised how the sensations change over the days or weeks. This is especially true for women in different phases of their menstrual cycle but applies to men too.

When you are well under way with this part of Step One, extend your self-discovery exercises to include your genitals. Once again take care to ensure you are private, warm, relaxed and comfortable and that you will not be interrupted. Look at your genitals, feel them carefully and get out a book to identify the various parts if you are not sure what is what. Do not aim for arousal; simply look and learn. You can then start to build up a sensuality profile of your genitals so that you become aware of the best parts and those that do not do much for you. If you are really keen you might want to do a little chart of these findings. Once you are completely happy with all of this you will be ready for the next step.

STEP TWO: GET TO KNOW YOUR PARTNER'S BODY AND GENITALS

This is much more difficult than Step One because it seems somewhat strange to go back to basic building blocks such as these with someone you may have known for many years. It is time well spent, however, so stay with it.

Take it in turns, one person per session, to explore one another's body in some detail. Keep away from breasts and genitals and avoid arousal at first or this will get in the way of your discovery. Share what you find and tenderly end your sessions with a kiss and a cuddle.

When you have completed this to your satisfaction make some private time to take it in turns to examine one another's genitals in some detail. I say 'in some detail' because many couples to whom I have suggested this over the years come back to their next therapy session having glimpsed one another's genitals for thirty seconds in failing light. They have clearly learned little or nothing from the exercise. Give yourselves a quarter of an hour to perform this task on just one of you. Work your way around all the parts, feeling as you go and using a book, if necessary, to identify parts of which you are unsure.

In a man you should be able to see the head of the penis and its slit-like opening that lets urine and semen out; the shaft of the penis with its few hairs and many veins; the balls in their sac, the scrotum; the root of the penis which runs from the base of the organ down towards the man's bottom; the area, between this and his anus; and the anus itself. When it comes to feeling, try to familiarize yourself with what is inside the various parts you can see and generally feel your way around the area, finding out what your partner likes best.

On a woman, start by looking at the large and small lips either side of the vulva; part these to display the little knob-like clitoris at the top and the hole that is the vagina below. Beneath this is the bridge of tissue called the perineum and further back the anus. Feel all these structures between finger and thumb; feel for the body of the clitoris, which is a pencil-like rod above the head of the organ towards the woman's tummy; and finally insert a finger into the vagina and see what the walls feel like. If you push your finger in further still you might be able to touch a tip-of-the-nose-like object which is her cervix, or opening to the womb.

You may not be able to achieve all this in one sitting so come back to it another day and try again. Really take your time. Try to take a pleasure in what you see and then talk to your partner about what you find interesting, surprising, or whatever. I have long since stopped being

surprised by couples who expect to enjoy a wonderfully fulfilling sexual and intimate life together and yet have never done any of this simple exploration. In a sense it is rather like wanting to enjoy the pleasures of motoring without ever have taken the trouble to learn where the controls of the car are.

So far none of our exercises in this section has included any kind of arousal. Should it occur by chance, the one who is aroused should take responsibility for relieving him or herself because at this stage it is wisest not to get involved in producing or taking responsibility for your partner's excitement. This will come in time but there are other stages to negotiate first.

STEP THREE: SENSUAL MASSAGE

This type of massage focuses on the giving and receiving of pleasure without producing sexual arousal. The key practical considerations are to ensure that you are relaxed and private; that the room is warm; and that you have some pleasant massage oil to work with. There are many books about this sort of massage but I have found, both personally and professionally, that the best thing to do is to follow your instincts, once you have mastered some very basic techniques.

At the heart of sensual massage is the implied goal of giving pleasure to our partner using only the hands. Listen carefully at first to what your partner says he or she enjoys best and make it your sole task to ensure that this pleasure is maximized. Slowly, after some sessions, you will become so adept at reading the slightest noise or body movement that you will completely do away with speaking and will still be able accurately to read your partner's bodily and internal responses.

After quite a lot of practice you may find that the whole experience becomes somewhat spiritual as you tune into one another's body at a very deep level – far more so than can be accounted for by touch alone. At this level sensual massage becomes a kind of meditation on your partner's body and you not only give but also receive in the process.

Experience shows that it is best either to give or receive a massage in any single session, rather than trying to do both. Taking it in turns session by session can be too slavish but be sure that if you are the 'giver' in your relationship generally (see page 52) you do not miss out on learning how to receive. I find that few people, once having surrendered to the sheer selfish pleasures of receiving are willing, or indeed able, to turn the tables and start to give at that same session.

As will be clear by now, I consider sensual massage to be far more than simply an exchange of 'nice touching'. The very act of being so open, trusting, naked and vulnerable is deeply symbolic in any relationship. The level of trust required is high and the opportunity for a sharing of souls is correspondingly great. Of all the physical techniques I teach my couples in therapy this is almost always rated as the most significant step towards intimacy. The agreement is that arousal is off the agenda; that the pleasure of the receiver is paramount; that his or her body be treated with respect; and that whatever is requested is given with an open heart. Couples have been telling me for years that this exercise alone makes vast inroads into intimacy. Courtship and other caring behaviour seem to flow from it; rows are fewer; and for the couple not having sex, massage alone can bring them closer together than they had ever felt possible.

STEP FOUR: LEARN HOW TO MASTURBATE

Although many people see masturbation as a somewhat adolescent or immature pastime in which one should not indulge in when in a loving, adult relationship, I have found that this attitude harms more people than it helps. Masturbation is, in fact, a vital part of most people's sexual life. I always say that masturbation is to sexual intercourse what talking is to debating.

This is no place to go into the pros and cons of masturbation but suffice it to say that we all have to be able to take responsibility for our own sexuality. I constantly see couples who blame and punish one another for not doing or being something sexual for them when in reality they have never learned to take responsibility for themselves. Just because we marry or embark on a long-term one-to-one relationship does not mean that we can give up on ourselves and hand over all future sexual arousal to our partner. It would be rather like expecting our loved one to feed us for the rest of our lives.

The vast majority of males have masturbated by the time they pair-bond with their lover and most continue to do so irrespective of how happy they are in their one-to-one relationship. The situation is slightly different for females because a somewhat larger proportion of them have not masturbated, or at least not consciously, before they finally settle down with a man. It is also my clinical experience that fewer women masturbate after marriage, or at least with any great frequency, than men do. The reasons for this are beyond the scope of this book.

Having said all this, it is my view that we cannot have an intimate relationship at a sexual level unless we can pleasure *ourselves* reliably. At the very simplest level it puts unnatural strains on the partnership if all sexual release has to come about through joint activities. The efforts of millions of couples to do this and the severe cost of failure bear out this claim in bedrooms all over the world every day. Masturbation without guilt or shame can be a difficult, or even impossible, task for some. I maintain, however, that unless this hurdle is somehow overcome, the same unconscious beliefs, fears or whatever that inhibit masturbation also plague the sexual and emotional union between ourselves and our partner, however subtly.

Begin by making your surroundings as relaxing and erotic as you can. Most of my patients say that it greatly helps to use some sort of erotic input such as a raunchy story, magazine, film or video. Women today, and especially younger ones, find all this much more acceptable than their mothers' generation did. Once you start to become aroused, experiment with your favourite types of genital play until you can reliably and happily produce orgasms for yourself. At this stage of sexual growth I find that it is helpful for men to teach themselves to slow down their arousal and progress towards orgasm and for women to learn to speed things up. This does not mean that on all subsequent sexual occasions the woman should come very quickly and the man very slowly but that each has more control, which they can then use to pleasure themselves, their partner, or both, depending on the mood of the particular session. You will find that this matching of your sexual tempos is difficult to learn during intercourse. It is far better achieved, initially, on your own. Taking responsibility for our own arousal is at the heart of any truly intimate sexual relationship.

Sensual massage can be an enduring tool in any couple's life together. Perhaps its greatest value is in being able to separate sexual intercourse from sensual touch, something many couples find difficult.

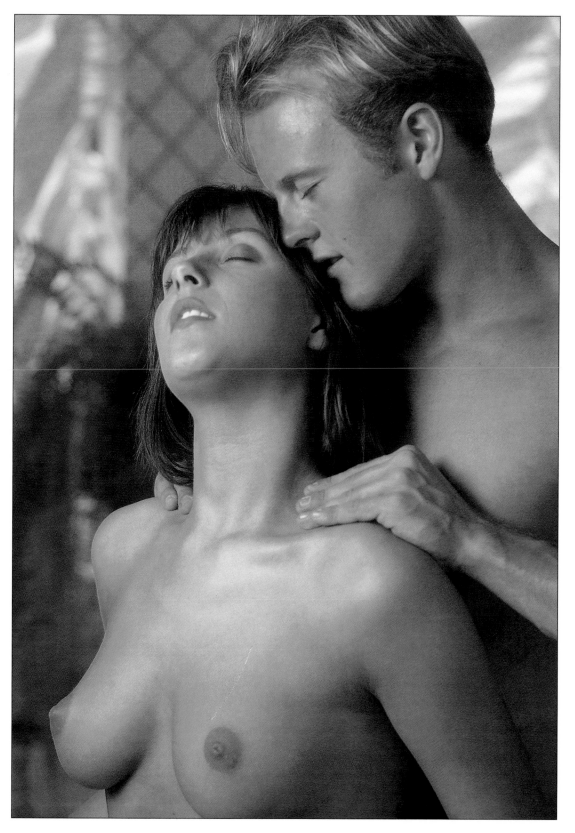

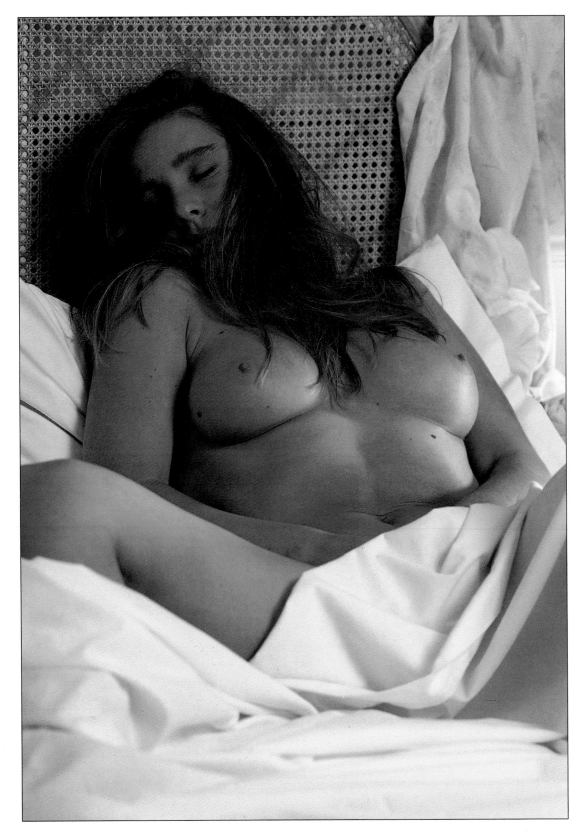

STEP FIVE: MASTURBATE IN FRONT OF YOUR PARTNER

A logical, if somewhat difficult, extension to Step Four is to take things further and to masturbate in front of your partner. This is usually much more demanding for women than for men but there are many shy men who have problems with it too.

Set the scene, as for all these private and 'risky' exercises. Agree who will go first and then one of you masturbate in front of the other. If you are shy, start off with the lights very dim, or even off, and then slowly, over some sessions, increase the light level until you are happy to have a climax in full view of your lover.

Be prepared for your orgasms to be and feel slightly different at first until you get used to being watched. If you find the presence of your partner too intimidating early on, arouse yourself as you normally would but with your partner out of the room, calling him or her in at the last moment as you approach orgasm. Whether or not you want to be touched, held, watched or whatever as you arouse yourself will be up to you and will probably change as time goes by. Take things gently if you are new to all this and see how it goes.

I know many readers will think this strange but what I tell my patients is that they should, perhaps after several such sessions, be able to give a highly detailed 'report' on their partner's arousal. This is not of academic interest – none of us is doing a Ph.D on our partner's sexuality. What matters is that by taking this much trouble really to learn and observe we become highly sensitive to our partner's arousal cycle and can then make this knowledge work to our advantage in our love-making. Many, if not most, men tell me that they have no idea what stage their partner is at in her arousal when they are making love. This disables them when it comes to pacing their own stimulation or their stimulation of her. It is astonishing that many couples who have been together for years have no idea how to read one another in bed. This can be speedily remedied by using this exercise.

Before we can be freely intimate sexually with our lover we have to know our own body and its responses. This can only be achieved by learning how to masturbate without guilt, fear or shame. This is very personal 'homework'.

Over some sessions you should both be able to sense, by direct and indirect methods, where each of you is in your journey through loveplay; how and if you are progressing towards orgasm; whether orgasm is in fact necessary or desirable; and so on. This work is hugely rewarding as it takes us deeper into our knowledge, experience and understanding of our lover as a unique human sexual being, not just as yet another member of the opposite sex.

STEP SIX: LEARN HOW TO MASTURBATE ONE ANOTHER

Knowing what you now know about your own arousal and that of your partner you are in a position to learn how to produce the very best possible sensations for him or her. This almost always means that the 'receiver' has gently to guide the 'giver' but you will be adept at this by now after all the practice you have had with sensual massage (see page 143). This is one of the situations where skills learned there begin to pay dividends.

A word of caution. Most people, when setting out on this exercise, find that they start telling their partner off if they do not get things right at once. Although it is extremely annoying to have someone do things wrongly in this respect, the best policy is gently but firmly to tell your partner what it is that you *do* want and lovingly to guide his or her efforts, rather than delivering a reprimand. Men in our culture are exceptionally sensitive about being 'corrected', as they see it, especially if they think they have considerable previous experience with other women. Sometimes the biggest risk of all is to open oneself up to doing this exercise in a relationship that has been working well for many years. To be gently guided to do something quite different from what we have become used to doing can feel threatening as the implication is that we have been getting it wrong for years. The thing to remember here is that you are best friends, not adversaries. Even a very long-term relationship can benefit from a sexual audit from time to time. If we are prepared to listen and learn *we* are the ones who gain. If we become defensive or offensive everyone loses.

I always challenge my couples to carry out this exercise on the basis that they should be able to end up masturbating their partner as well as their partner can masturbate himself or herself, and probably even better. In fact many individuals say that, however good their own self-pleasuring, it is always different and usually better when their lover does it.

If you want to take this a stage further you could now start to masturbate one another at the same time, learning how to postpone the delights of orgasm or speed them up at will. The confidence that this builds and the level of trust and intimacy that results has to be experienced to be believed.

STEP SEVEN: SHARE YOUR FANTASIES

The sharing of fantasies is one of the major building blocks of true sexual intimacy. It calls for considerable levels of trust; for acceptance of our lover for himself or herself, whatever we think about the fantasy. It helps us celebrate our partner's difference from us, (see page 133), which is partly why we love this person. It can open us up to parts of ourselves and our own sexuality that we would otherwise have kept hidden; and much more.

Sharing fantasies is, however, a tricky issue that should be taken cautiously. Just because we have a fantasy does not mean that we ought to share it 'because it shows how I really am and you ought to know'. Quite the contrary, in my experience. Many fantasies should *never* be shared but only you will know what feels safe and respectful of your own particular relationship. Real no-nos are those fantasies that involve people you both know personally. Many individuals, women especially, fear that such fantasies could become fact given half a chance. Only very trusting and experienced lovers with a great depth of intimacy in the rest of their lives can deal with fantasies that contain high levels of 'threatening' material. Being 'sexually together' on the subject of sex in general is usually not enough.

Begin by sharing simple and inoffensive fantasies, perhaps after seeing something at the cinema or on a video. Some couples use sexy magazines to feed this sort of exploration. An exercise that works well is for both to write a one-page script (on separate sheets of paper) that could form the basis for an XXX-rated video. Then swap them. You will be surprised how much you can learn about your partner's most intimate fantasy life.

Whether or not you end up acting out any of your shared fantasies will be up to you but it is best to start off by agreeing that sharing puts neither of you under any obligation to *do* any-

thing about them. Most of us have paired for very good unconscious reasons (see page 35) so it is not at all uncommon for couples who have never shared fantasies to find that they either have very similar ones or that they are highly complementary and match one another very well. This is the sort of unconscious business that brought the couple together in the first place as they unknowingly sought to heal themselves.

I hope I have made it clear that sharing fantasies is not a sort of party game, although of course it can be huge fun and can open up our sexual lives in ways that few other activities can. As well as all this, however, the sharing of fantasies can, if done against the background of an intimate relationship, give insights into ourselves and our partner that are near-impossible to gain outside some sort of formal therapy.

STEP EIGHT: EROTIC MASSAGE

This is a way of touching one another that, unlike sensual massage, is specifically geared to producing sexual arousal. The erotic opportunities that are open to you by using your hands, nails, hair, body, genitals, toys, materials, foods and so on is limited only by your imagination and your unconscious inhibitions. By this stage I hope the latter will be well on the way out of your lives as a result of the intimacy and trust that is growing between you.

This is the time to let your dreams run wild, to try anything that appeals to either of you and to break new ground, especially if you have been in a sexual rut for some years. This sort of massage usually ends in love-making.

STEP NINE: LOVE-MAKING

I hope that by this stage you will be aware of the distinction I draw between 'having sex' and 'making love' (see page 98). It can be fun and highly arousing occasionally to let ourselves go, to be spontaneous and to enjoy one another at a purely carnal level. This sort of sex, however, does not appeal to many as a staple diet.

Love-making, in the way that I am describing it, is personalized to our partner; is as much partner-centred as it is self-centred; reinforces our

---

The sharing and acting out of fantasies should be done with great care. Getting your partner to help feed your fantasy can turn an ordinary session into a magical one.

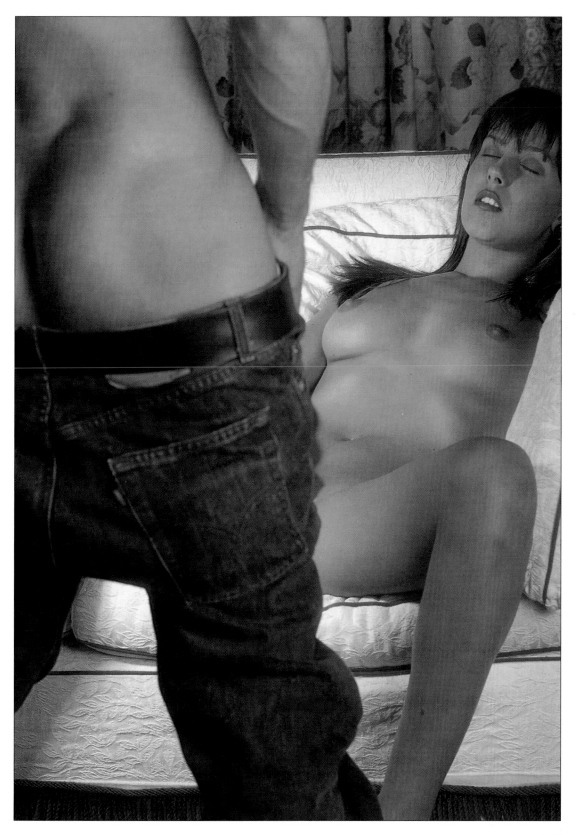

commitment to each other; involves our genitals as part of our whole personality; is a mutually co-operative activity; calls for insight and imagination; improves with time; enhances the value of our partner to us; has limitless horizons; adapts well to occasional failure; implies a policy of continuous improvement; and is a lifetime's investment. Quite a list.

None of this is possible without intimacy. Perhaps this is why so many people, and especially males in our culture, are constantly complaining about 'not having enough sex'. I think most have more than enough 'sex' but far too few make love in the way I have described here. In therapy I often tell couples that I am going to get them to have *less* sex. At first they think I am joking but as it becomes clear to them that what I mean is more high-quality love-making and less loveless copulation, they soon see how appealing the suggestion is.

STEP TEN: SHARE TAKING THE LEAD

The last stage in the growth of sexual intimacy involves working on your ability to share the 'control' issues that arise in your sexual life. Many couples tell me that they have a wonderful time in bed but that something they cannot identify is missing. As we have seen throughout the book this 'something' is often intimacy, even if the couple is close, friendly, erotic and so on. There are many couples, however, who live out the same sexual scenario year after year, acting largely out of old unconscious scripts that say that men ought to do X and women Y in bed. All the love in the world will not heal the anger, disappointment, frustration and fear that such beliefs can produce in a vulnerable partner. We may feel we have to act out a cultural stereotype, (in other words we might do so because we have conscious control and choose to accept the model); or we might do so for perfectly unconscious reasons that hurt our partner, ourselves, or both of us.

Being able to exchange 'control' in sex so that either partner is able to take the initiative helps build sexual intimacy very powerfully. It is, in fact, impossible to have come this far in this book and do otherwise. As soon as we pigeonhole our partner as 'a woman' or 'a man' we lose sight of them as a whole human being who might exhibit all kinds of masculine and feminine colourations within his or her personality structure. Just because I am a male does not mean that the caring, soft and gentle 'feminine'

side of my personality cannot come out to play when making love. The reverse is true for a woman. Many of us can find our opposite-sex psychic twin from within the recesses of our unconscious *only* in the safety, trust and regressive love of our sexual encounters.

If anything significant is taking place in the world of man-woman relationships today it is perhaps that males are more able to accept and exhibit their 'feminine' characteristics while still being seen as truly 'male'. The reverse has to some extent been happening for far longer with females as the women's movement over the last thirty years has enabled females of all ages to embrace such concepts in theory and practice. When men can fully accept and revel in their feminine side and when their partners can do the same for their masculine principle perhaps we shall redress the imbalance that so many men feel has occurred in this respect over the last generation. Many men tell me that they quite envy their wife who is free to be a feminine woman and also to acknowledge and benefit from the more masculine side of her personality at work and in the home. Somehow we, as a society, have become so absorbed in this that we have overlooked men's desire to express their opposite-sex polarity too. Most men's fears of being labelled homosexual or 'like a woman' prevent them from celebrating their femininity and incorporating it within their otherwise perfectly acceptable masculinity.

Once men can incorporate this feminine principle they will then be all the better equipped to become 'real men' again. Most women I listen to say that modern men have lost something. Whether Robert Bly in his book *Iron John* has identified it by asserting that men should become more healthily 'fierce', developing their 'inner warrior' from a position not of aggression or hostility but from the soul of the 'wild man' within, only time will tell. From where I sit every day, some sort of return to a celebration of the differences between men and women whilst also accepting the similarities, is the best start towards a healthy growth of sexual intimacy.

Now that you have enhanced your sexual and bedroom intimacy you may be interested in three final exercises that will call for all your new-found skills. The goodwill and fun that you have created in purely sexual matters should now enable you to tackle some of the most tricky areas on your journey: no-go areas, forgiveness and fun.

— EXERCISE ELEVEN —

NO-GO AREAS

In every relationship there are subjects that are hardly ever addressed because they bring heartache or worse when they are. These I call 'no-go areas'. We all have them but problems arise when we do not recognize them.

For reasons of which we are largely unaware, we all have set attitudes concerning every possible area of life. Whether it is the way children should be educated; oral sex; who should be in charge of family finances; women and work; breast-feeding, or whatever, each of us has a unique position, whether it is held in our conscious, unconscious or a mixture of the two.

There are bound to be areas of life on which we cannot agree. In good, working relationships such matters are often amicably settled by negotiation. In certain zones of life, however, the no-go areas, issues remain unmentioned for years on end because we fear the risk involved in raising them at all.

That no-go areas are common is no great tragedy in itself and certainly no fatal barrier to intimacy. This is rarely all there is to it, however. Most of find that over the years together our no-go areas not only proliferate but grow in size so that after, say, ten years together old ones are so entrenched that they do not permit even occasional airing and new ones are grafted on to them. This makes almost any in-depth discussion seem dangerous for fear of hitting on a no-go area or one of its extensions.

Couples living like this, and millions do, find that they only ever communicate at the most superficial level about almost everything. To behave in any other way is to lay themselves open to the minefield that is their cumulative no-go zone. Eventually they can talk about almost nothing and the relationship dies.

I have left the subject of no-go areas till this late stage in the journey towards intimacy because it takes formidable skills to traverse such a minefield. I have found, too, that most people benefit hugely from developing the sorts of abilities outlined in this section and from an enriched sexual life before they embark on this difficult area. The amount of goodwill generated by better sex and increased intimacy enables even very dangerous no-go areas to be tackled.

How you decide to do this will be up to you.

By this stage in your journey you will have discovered how you best deal with highly charged emotional issues and you will be really good at listening to one another empathically. A good place to start is for each of you to make a list of subjects that are out of bounds. Some of these will seem relatively unimportant and could remain as 'non-issues' for some time. There are, however, always one or two major no-go zones in every partnership that are well worth airing, provided that this can be done safely.

A way that I find works well for many people is to agree on a couple of topics each. For example, she might raise 'my job once the children leave home' and 'your demands for oral sex'; and he might want to deal with 'the affair you had five years ago' and '*my* bad feelings towards *your* mother'. I have found that many people are unable to discuss such topics from cold so I usually suggest that they write down the main points that they *feel* about the topic. When doing this include as many 'I' statements as possible and keep things focused on yourself. Try, with the knowledge gained from all the work you have done, to put these feelings into some sort of context within your family of origin. Then write a short paragraph or two that summarizes all this.

When you feel the time is right and you have an opportunity to talk it through, show your partner your writing and give him or her time alone to think about it. Perhaps leave things for a few days before you actually talk. This will give your partner a chance to chew over the subject; to think about what is behind what you are actually saying and feeling; to formulate some responses if the no-go area affects him or her personally; and generally allow some level of healing and understanding to occur.

When it comes to discussing things, set a time limit; remember to listen as much as you talk; do not forget that your partner is probably your best friend; and at the end create a list of thoughts or actions on which you both agree and write them down. The magnitude of the issues in a no-go area often becomes amplified over the months or years and what initially looked like an unclimbable mountain can turn out to be a small hillock given some intimacy skills. Remember, as I have emphasized throughout the book, that there is no right or wrong in such discussions: usually you will both be right in your own ways. The level of intimacy that you will by now share

Continued on page 155

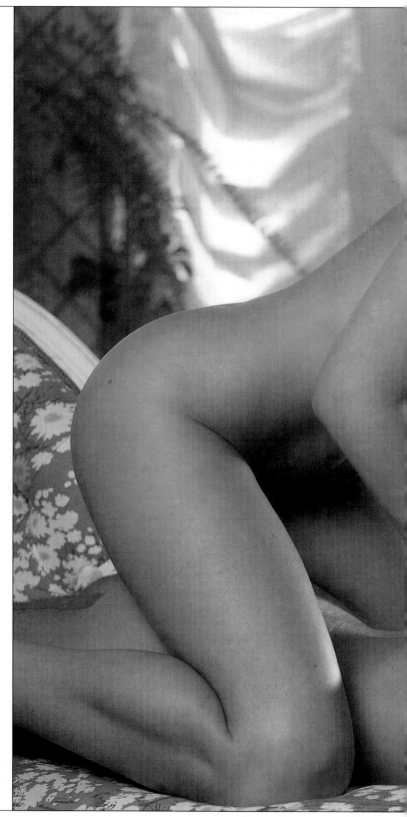

Erotic massage takes sensual play one step further to produce arousal actively. Anything goes, provided that it is personalized to our lover and is exactly what he or she best enjoys. The trust that exists between true intimates ensures that they both get the most out of the experience.

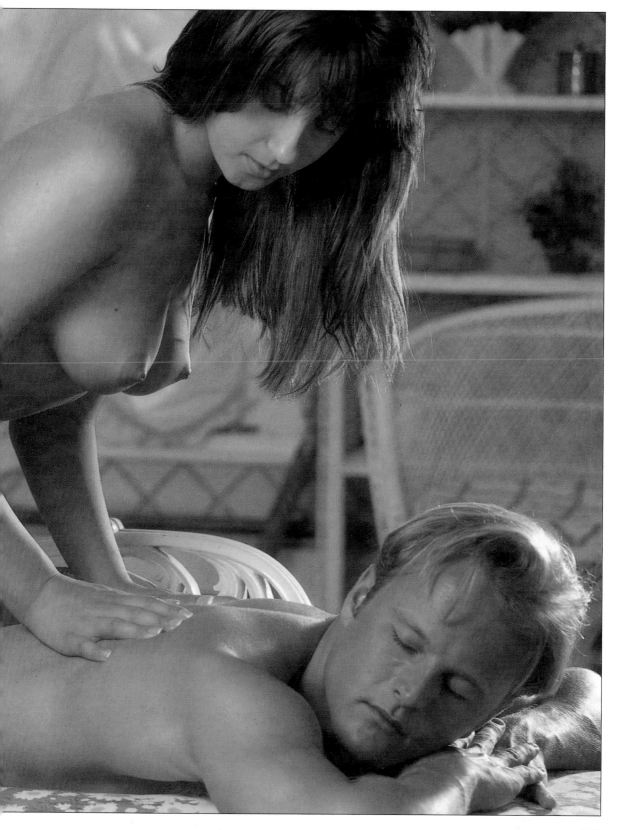

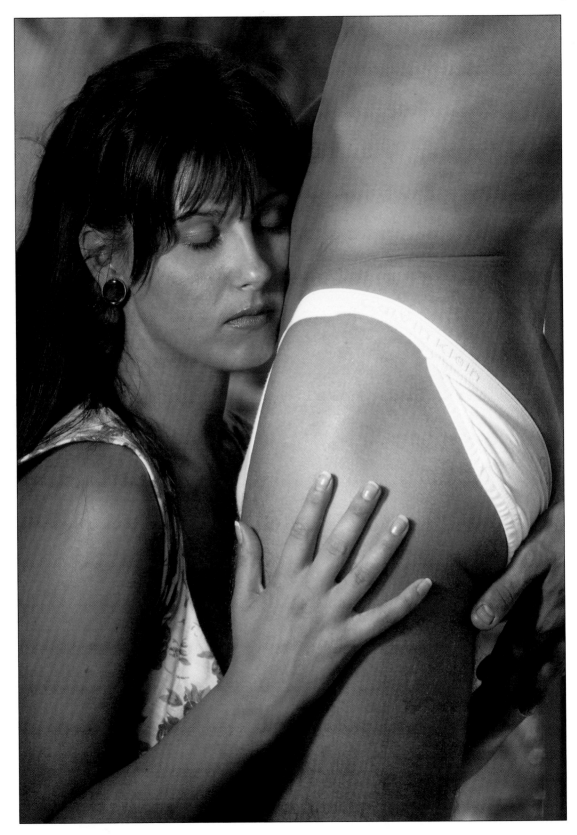

should allow you graciously to accept that your stubborn need always to be right (see page 80) has only served to increase the power of your no-go areas and that you might now, with some charm, be able to give up the struggle and walk alongside your partner as he or she battles it out in his or her own heart and soul. This sort of work often calls for the ability to forgive.

—————— EXERCISE TWELVE ——————
FORGIVENESS

This subject is covered in more depth on page 85 but here let me reiterate that most of us cannot 'forgive and forget' and nor should we. The mature individual is one who can forgive and remember.

One day, when you are on your own, think about what there is in your relationship that you need to forgive. Make a short list of the items in order to make them real to yourself. Next, describe and explain to yourself the things for which you need to *be* forgiven. When it comes to sharing all this with your partner it often helps to start the ball rolling with this latter part and to talk about an issue that does not involve him or her personally or both of you as a couple. Share between you whether you find it easier to forgive or to be forgiven. Perhaps read the section beginning on page 85 for ideas.

This exercise takes us into the very depths of ourselves, which is why I have left it to so near the end. Start with simple issues and, if you feel safe enough over the months, you might be able to tackle topics that have made you feel guilty, ashamed, or worse, for years or perhaps even for a whole lifetime. The freedom that such revelations bring changes people lives and undoubtedly alters relationships.

It is easy to love the lovable and forgive the forgivable. A deep and intimate relationship worthy of its name somehow enables us to love the unlovable and forgive the unforgivable in ourselves and our partner. This touching of souls is usually reflected in the whole of our lives and for

Sharing taking the lead in love-making is a sign of a mature relationship between equals. In such a couple neither 'does' things to the other and both are free to be passive or active from time to time.

many couples creates a freedom in sex that they had never previously found possible. Removing old guilt, fear and shame, and feeling truly forgiven by oneself, one's partner, or both now frees us to embark on the last exercise on our journey.

—————— EXERCISE THIRTEEN ——————
PLAY AND FUN

Apart from many of the purely sexual exercises, most of the activities I have described in Part Three have been somewhat serious. Having said this, many people find that even when they are dealing with weighty matters they can still have a laugh. Indeed as a therapist I find myself having many a laugh with my patients. It is said that laughter is the best medicine and there is certainly more than a grain of truth in this. Inside everyone is a childlike part that craves to be heard. How we let our inner child out to play is unique to each one of us. Some people rarely do so and lead very serious lives either as individuals or as couples.

Although you could, of course, use this exercise at any point in your journey I have left it till last because in a way it is the crowning glory of a really intimate relationship. Couples that can be sufficiently themselves to feel free enough to let their inner little child out to play are well on the way to where they want to be on their intimate journey together.

Draw up separate lists of fun things that you would like to do with your partner. They must be one-to-one pastimes that involve only your partner. They can be mental or physical. Some examples of what I mean are: tickling; wrestling; making love; throwing him or her into the swimming pool; having a bath together; cycling; playing a board game; seeing a show; watching an X-rated video; and so on. Put both your lists together and choose one new activity to do per week for the near future. Make sure that you balance out choices from one another's lists.

Many couples find it difficult to do silly things together and to let their inner child out to play. You might even find that your own children are resistant to you doing what they think are silly things. Stick with it. Ignore everyone but yourselves and get back to uninhibited fun both in and out of bed. I generally have an aversion to simplistic aphorisms, but 'The couple that plays together stays together' is not too awful!

MAKING IT HAPPEN

When I first explain to couples in therapy what the journey towards intimacy involves some of them claim that any such programme will be nearly impossible for them to implement because they are simply too busy. My answer is that we can always find time for something that we really want to do. Indeed the majority of those with whom I deal end up making the time. This means making your journey towards greater intimacy a major priority, if only for a few months while you get your teeth into some real progress. After this you will probably find that you can afford to coast along and still maintain the kind of intimate life you both want.

Early on, however, you will need to make time for the exercises. I have found both in my own life and in those of my patients that this can best be achieved by creating some sort of schedule in which to do things together. Many couples find that they need to dedicate an evening a week to this work and so never book themselves up for anything at this time. This not only ensures that they actually have time set aside to achieve something of worth but also gives the keener one in the partnership, and there is always one who wants to do this work more than the other, the confidence that things will not just slip. We are all somewhat lazy and it is easy to allow even the best intentions to wither on the bough as other tasks and activities in life appear to be more important. Setting aside a special time can mean staying at home; going out for a simple meal together; spending an evening in a pub; going for a walk or drive; and so on. Many couples tell me that the womb-like nature of a car can make for meaningful sharing.

Whilst all this formality might appear rather neurotic to the average reader, most couples in my experience find it difficult to create space for themselves to carry out this sort of relationship growth and servicing and have to plan it very thoughtfully. This is especially true for couples with young children.

As time goes by and you become really adept at intimate sharing you will probably find that you can carry out such business in informal settings that would have been unthinkable when you were starting out. This all comes about by trial and error in most relationships that work. It is rather like learning to drive. At first everything we do seems false and indeed it is. We then take the driving test and probably never drive like that again in our lives. After this, intuition takes over and most of us drive on autopilot. So it is with intimate relationships once we have the basic skills. We no longer have to think about listening empathically, for example, after a while. The same is true of bedroom intimacies. Thoughtful and loving work put in early on reaps huge rewards. Just as the pleasures of motoring become apparent when we forget the mechanics, so it is with intimacy.

The intimate couple grow together; fight together; make love together and usually stay together. All of this is a lifetime's journey and investment but it would be difficult to think of one that was more worthwhile.

No amount of head knowledge can make us intimate with our lover. It takes time, effort, understanding and goodwill. In short, we have to make it happen. For most of us this is one of life's greatest joys.

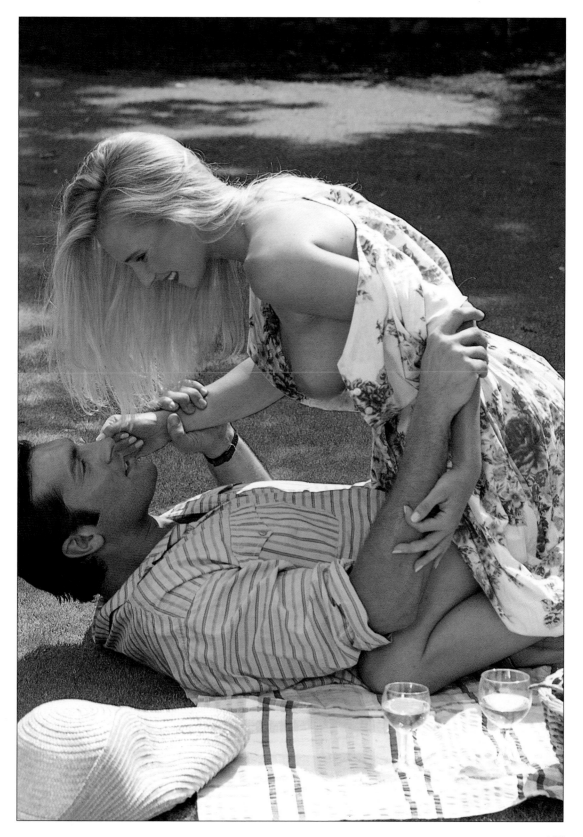

FURTHER READING

In addition to many learned papers from the psychological and medical literature, I have found the following books interesting in various different ways. Few of them deal directly with sexual intimacy but each adds something to the literature on the subject and can be read in different ways depending on your starting point.

Bach, George R. and Wyden, Peter. *The Intimate Enemy*,
New York, Avon Books, 1968

Crowther, C. Edward. *Intimacy — Strategies for Successful Relationships*,
New York, Dell Publishing, 1986

Emmons, L. and Alberti, R. *Accepting Each Other*,
San Luis Obispo, CA, Impact Publishers, 1991

Greenwald, Jerry. *Creative Intimacy*,
New York, Simon & Schuster, 1975

Lerner, Harriet Goldhor. *The Dance of Intimacy*,
New York, Harper and Row, 1989;
Wellingborough, Thorsons Publishers Limited, 1990

Malone, P. and T. *The Art of Intimacy*,
London, Simon & Schuster, 1987

Morris, Desmond. *Intimate Behaviour*,
New York, Random House, 1971

Powell, G. *Listening and Loving*,
Atlanta, Gleam Powell, 1985

Rubin, Lilian. *Intimate Strangers*,
New York, Harper and Row, 1984

Stanway, Dr Andrew. *The Art of Sensual Loving*,
London, Headline, 1989; New York, Carroll & Graf, 1989

Tannen, Deborah. *You Just Don't Understand*,
New York, William Morrow, 1988

Yorke, Andrew. *The Art of Erotic Massage*,
London, Cassell, 1988.

INDEX